I Call Him My Brother

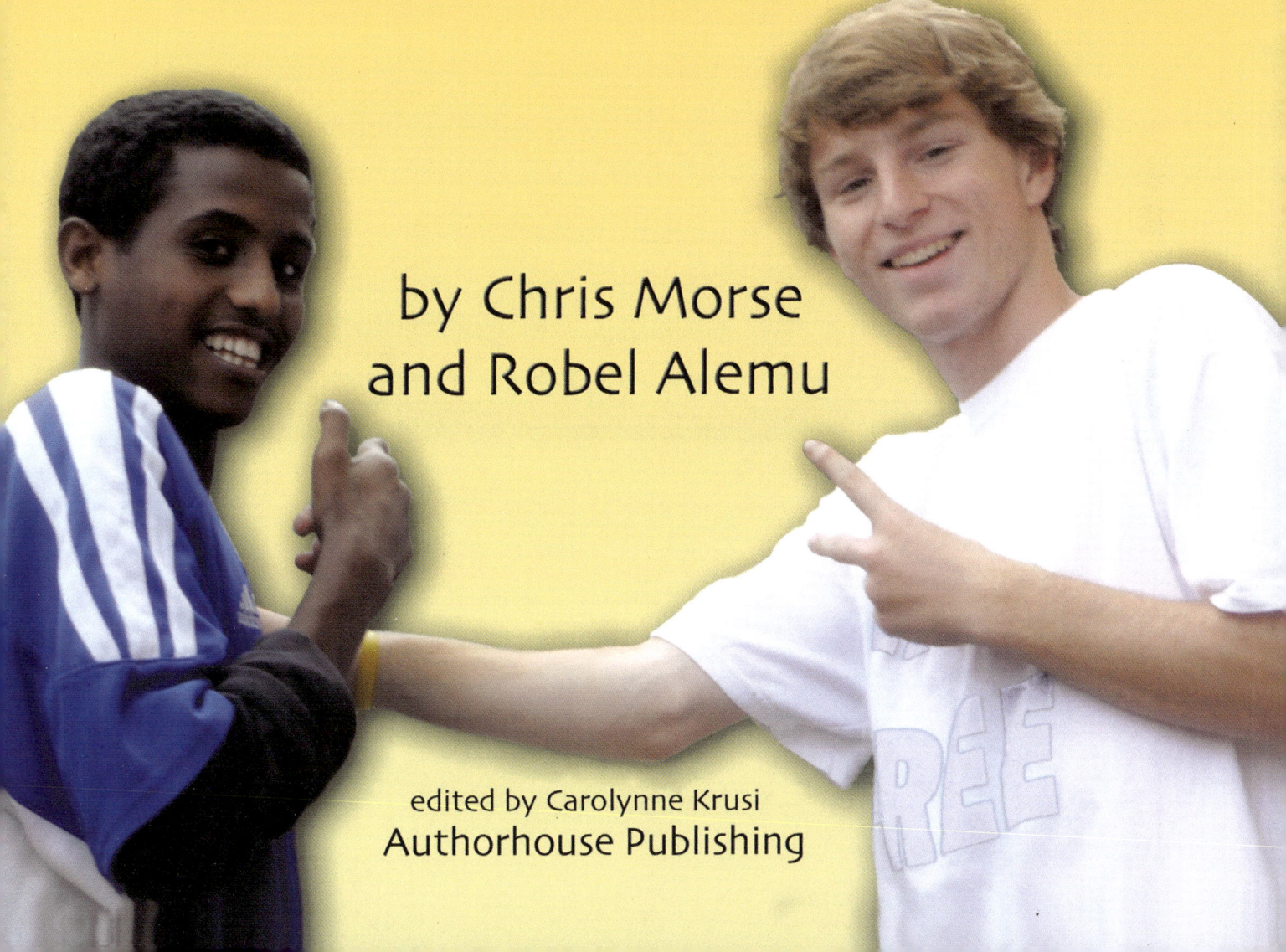

by Chris Morse
and Robel Alemu

edited by Carolynne Krusi
Authorhouse Publishing

Those who enjoy this book may also enjoy:

An Unlikely Family; Voices of Ethiopian and American Youth Who are Turning Tragedy into Hope.

The Selamta Family Project may be contacted at
802-649-7094
mia@selamtafamilyproject.org
http://www.selamtafamilyproject.org

SELAMTA
FAMILY PROJECT

©2012 by Selamta Family Project. All rights reserved. No part of this book may be reproduced, stored in a retrieval system, or transmitted by any means without the written permission of the authors.

Published by AuthorHouse 11/28/2012

ISBN 978-1-4343-6546-0 (sc)

This book is printed on acid-free paper.

Because of the dynamic nature of the Internet, any web addresses or links contained in this book may have changed since publication and may no longer be valid. The views expressed in this work are solely those of the author and do not necessarily reflect the views of the publisher, and the publisher hereby disclaims any responsibility for them.

AuthorHouse™
1663 Liberty Drive
Bloomington, IN 47403
www.authorhouse.com
Phone: 1-800-839-8640

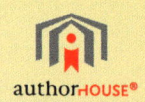

authorHOUSE®

Table of Contents

Acknowledgments and Dedication...................................4
Robel and Chris..6
Selamta..8
Getting to Selamta
   Chris 12
   Robel 14
Welcome to the Family 20
The Van..28
The Circus 32
To the Hospital 34
Futball (Soccer)..36
Inside Selamta Families 38
The Mercato..48
School 52
Entoto 54
Life on the Streets 62
A Special Dinner 78
Mekdes and Yeshi 80
Afterward...89
About Selamta 90

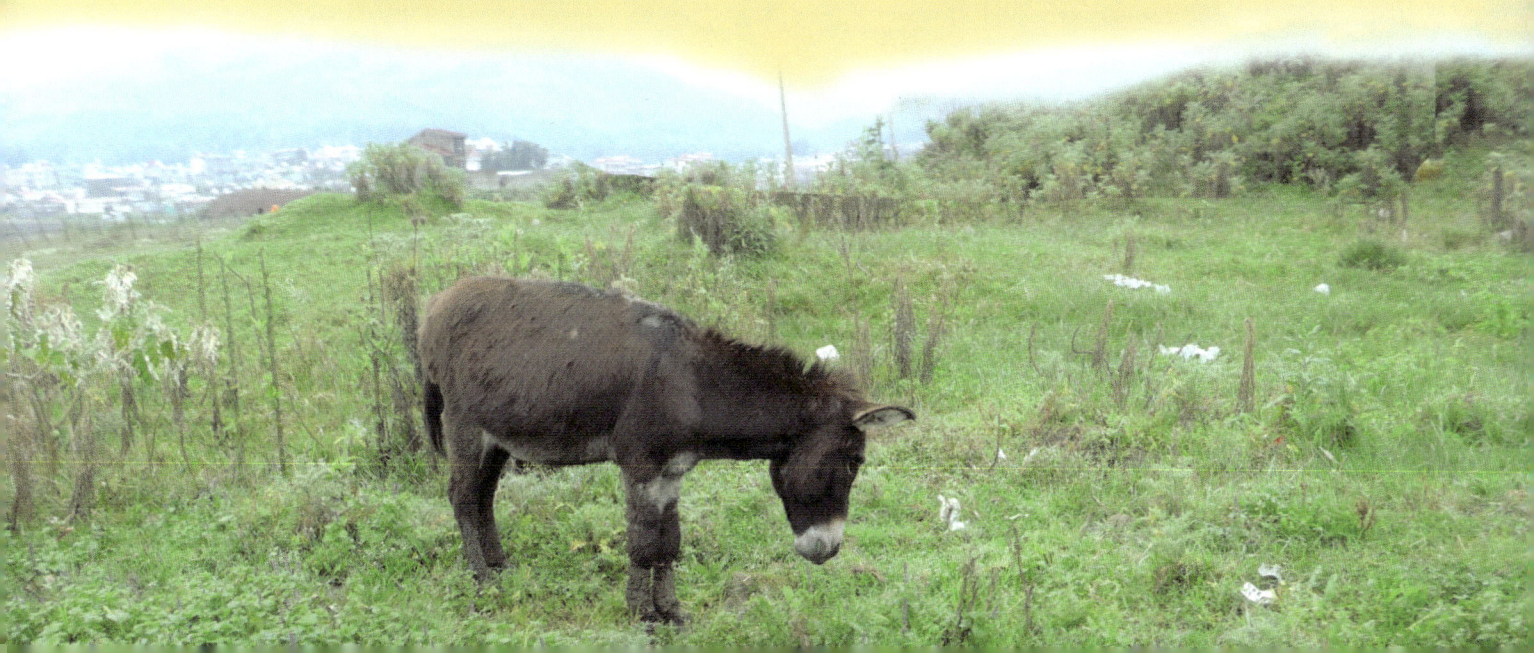

Special Acknowledgments

To Mia Brown for doing so much for the children of Selamta, both in the US and in Ethiopia, for joining us on our journeys, and for helping so much with the book.

To Abel Solomon who makes everything happen at Selamta.

To Esmael Atsedaw for being our friend, guide and translator, and for offering endless support.

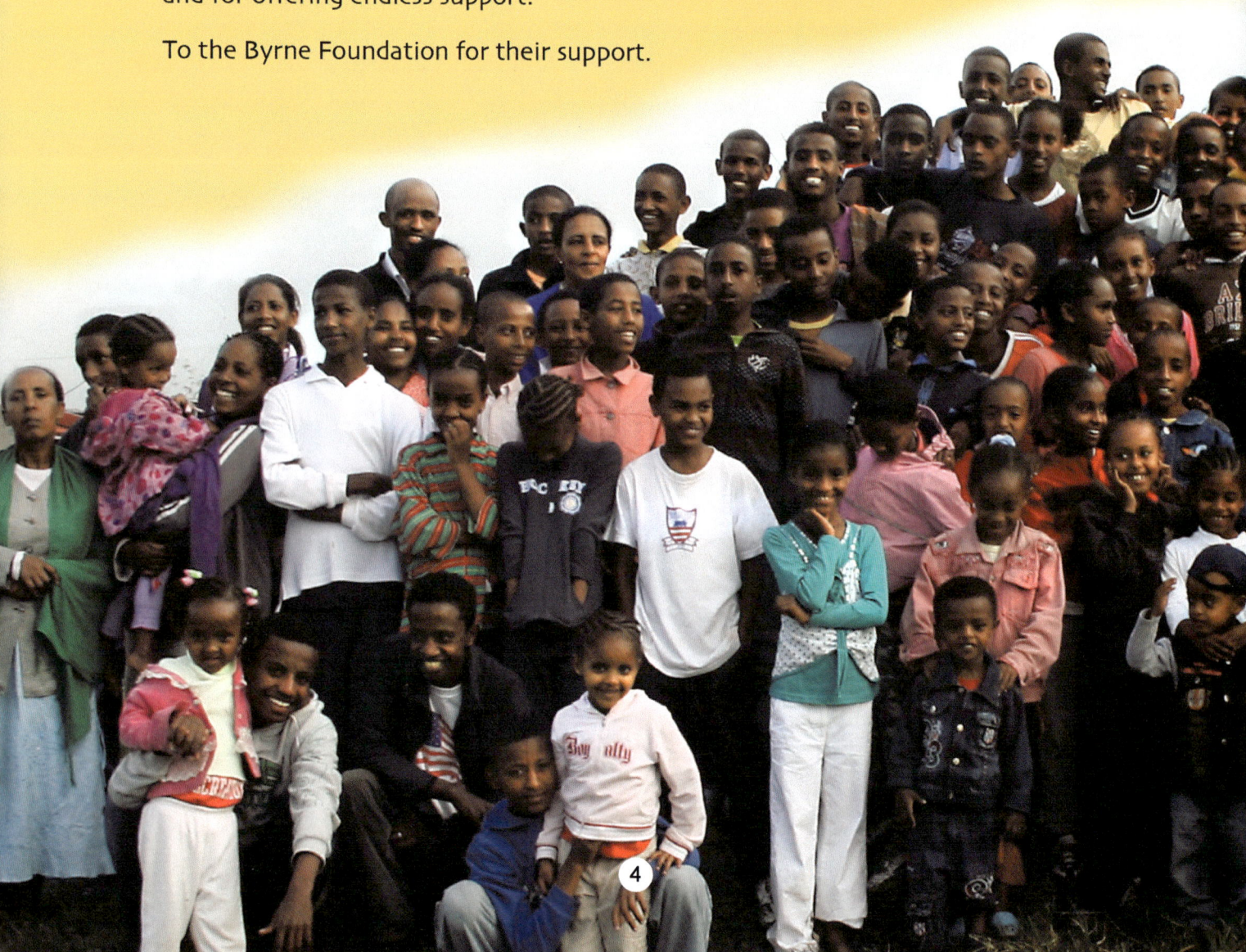

To the Byrne Foundation for their support.

Dedication

This book is dedicated to the Ethiopian children of Selamta who have found love within their new families, and to the three women called "angels" by these Selamta children: Carolynne Krusi, Bray Mitchell and Carol Foster.

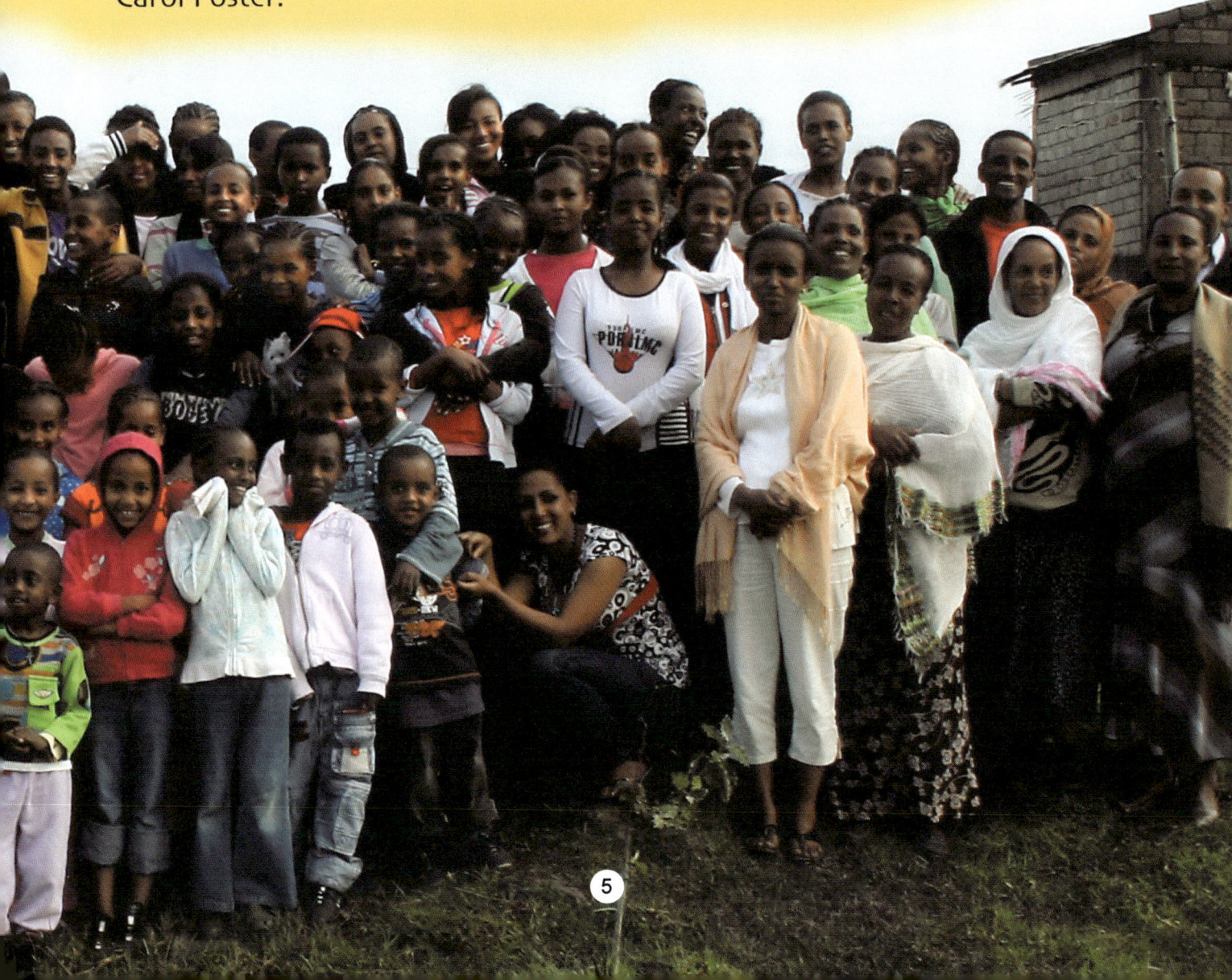

Robel

Age: 17 years old

Born: Buja, Ethiopia

Current Home:
With my new family in Addis Ababa, Ethiopia

Favorite Sport: Futball (Soccer)

Passion: Music

Goals for the Future:
For my work, I would like to help street children, and I also want to have a big workshop.
I hope to work in the mechanics field in the future. Maybe, besides being a singer and helping the children, I will build my own airplane or something like that. I like mechanics, things like planes and cars.

One wish:
If I have just one wish, my dream is to be a famous singer in Ethiopia like Teddy Afro.

Chris

Age: 18 years old

Born: Hanover, New Hampshire

Current Home:
Yale University, New Haven Connecticut

Favorite Sports: Lacrosse and Skiing

Favorite Pastime:
Spending time with my family and my dogs.

Goals for Future:
My goals are always changing, and molding into new and exciting possibilities. Given my New England background, the environment is extremely important to me. Working for renewable resources in less fortunate regions of the world excites me!

One wish: If I could have one wish, I hope for everyone to understand the challenges faced by millions of children world-wide every day, and that this would result in more compassion and aid for those with daily struggles.

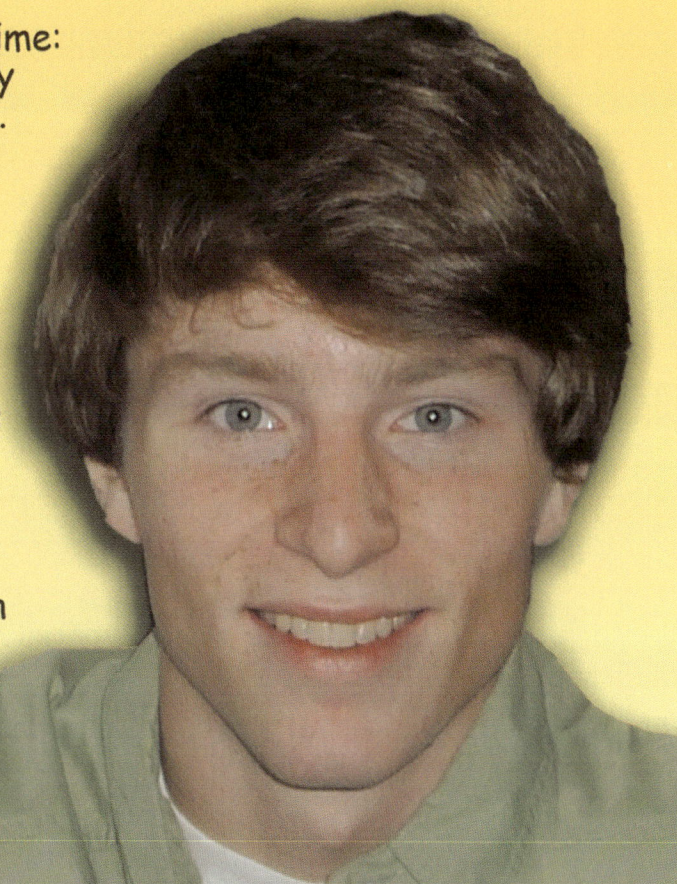

Selamta

Chris:

February 18, 2005

It all started on a cold New Hampshire February vacation day when I went to visit Tariku Foster, one of my friends from middle school. As I approached his front steps, I saw over twenty large jars filled to the brim with change. I thought it was pretty unusual that my friend would have all of these jars of seemingly insignificant change, but I didn't immediately ask him of their purpose.

Later, as Tariku and I were hanging out at his house, I tentatively approached the subject of the bottles full of change on the front porch. When I asked, he seemed genuinely interested in sharing his story.

It turns out that Tariku is one of seven adopted children making up the Foster family. He was adopted from Ethiopia, and his mom, Carol Foster, was starting an organization called the Selamta Family Project. Tariku told me that the jars were individual donations for this newly founded non-profit organization committed to creating new families for orphans in Addis Ababa, Ethiopia. At the time, I had no idea that this was an introduction to an organization that would change my life.

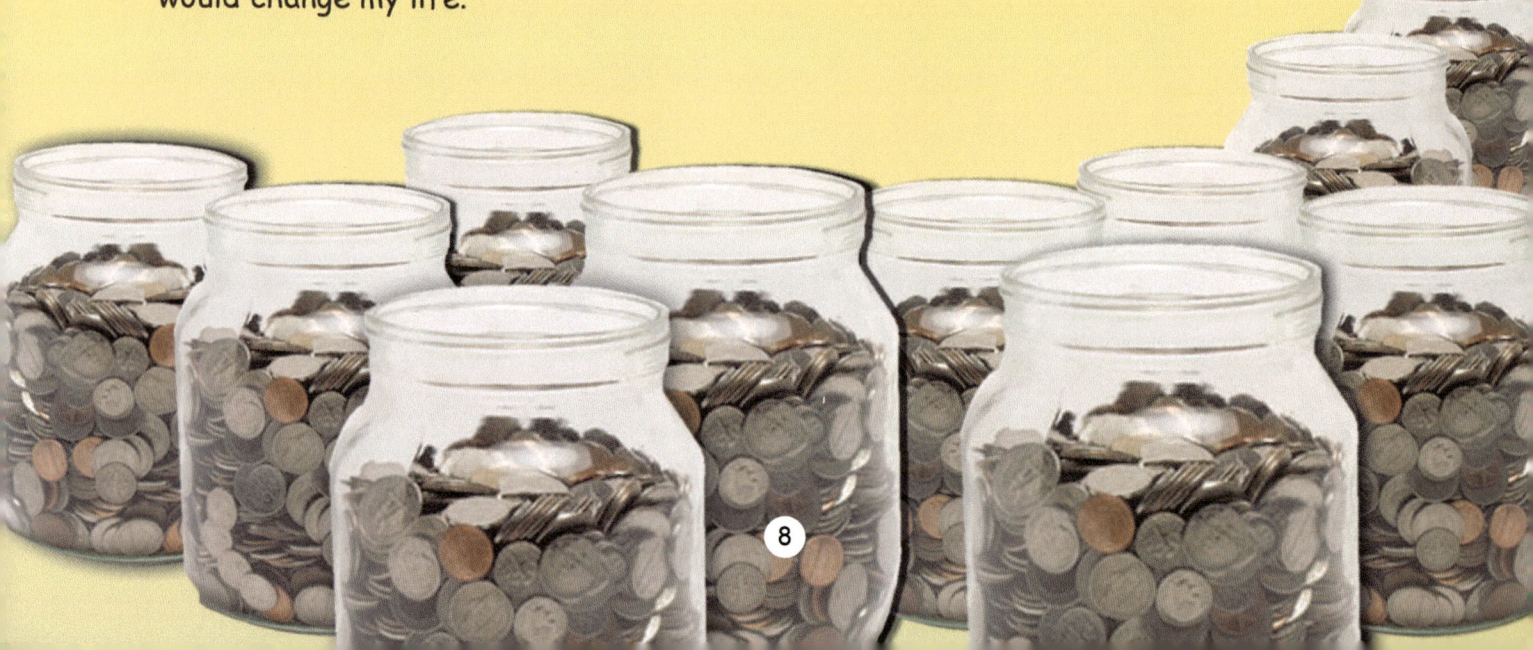

About The Selamta Family Project

The Selamta Children's Project in Addis Ababa, Ethiopia is a new, sustainable family model. HIV/AIDS has left millions of Ethiopian children orphaned, with women widowed and abandoned to the margins of society. The Selamta Family Project, a grassroots project developed in 2005, establishes permanent, stable family homes for these orphaned children and marginalized women. By providing positive influences in a family and community setting, it is possible to build strong citizens, maintain cultural connections, and sustain healthy conditions.

The Project offers a thorough training program for the women (child development, health, and household skills) who are chosen to become heads of new Selamta families. These new "mothers" along with eight to nine children form a new family. These families then move into a modern house painted and furnished by volunteers traveling to Ethiopia, along with the new family transforming it into a new home. These new families are permanent, and offer love, respect and safety.

Since the project began, there have been eleven homes created, over a hundred orphans placed into families, and twenty two women have become heads of households. All of the children attend school; many are on the honor roll. The soccer team is winning, and one hundred percent of the children are immunized. In other words, these children and their new mothers are thriving.

Selamta is not an orphanage, but a new life-start from the streets to a unique place within the Selamta Family and society. This model is successful in Ethiopia and is proving to be a sustainable model to re-incorporate women into society, children into families, and produce healthy citizens who are future leaders in their country.

Chris:

September 2009-August 2010
A Vision with a Lot of Work Attached

I wanted my junior year of high school to be memorable. In pursuit of opportunities to implement change, I remembered my introduction to the Selamta Family Project. I contacted the leaders of the organization, Carol Foster and Carolynne Krusi, and asked them what the children of Selamta needed. We met on numerous occasions, and they put me in touch with an Ethiopian boy my age, named Robel. Robel and I began corresponding, and from his stories, it became apparent that Selamta needed reliable transportation.

Currently, whenever transportation is needed, a costly taxi or gari (horse and carriage) is required, which takes away money that could be used in other ways for the children of Selamta. Also, relying on taxis takes valuable time because of the distance they must travel and the conditions of the roads.

I recognized that there was a clear need for a van for Selamta. With the help of Mrs. Foster and Ms. Krusi, I planned my fundraising activities.

Robel and I communicated over the course of the year, and we became friends as we shared the stories of our lives on different continents. Every time I would hear from Robel, I became even more determined to buy a van for Selamta. After nearly a year of planning, and a lot of local help, this became a reality. I scheduled a trip to Addis to coincide with the delivery of the new van.

When I first heard of Selamta and of its needs, I admit that the idea of raising money for a van that would be used in a city a world away from my home sounded daunting, if not ludicrous. The woods of New Hampshire share nothing in common with the streets of Addis. And yet, in this day and age, it's impossible not to be aware of the plight of the orphans in Africa. I was determined to find out what their lives were like and what I could do to help.

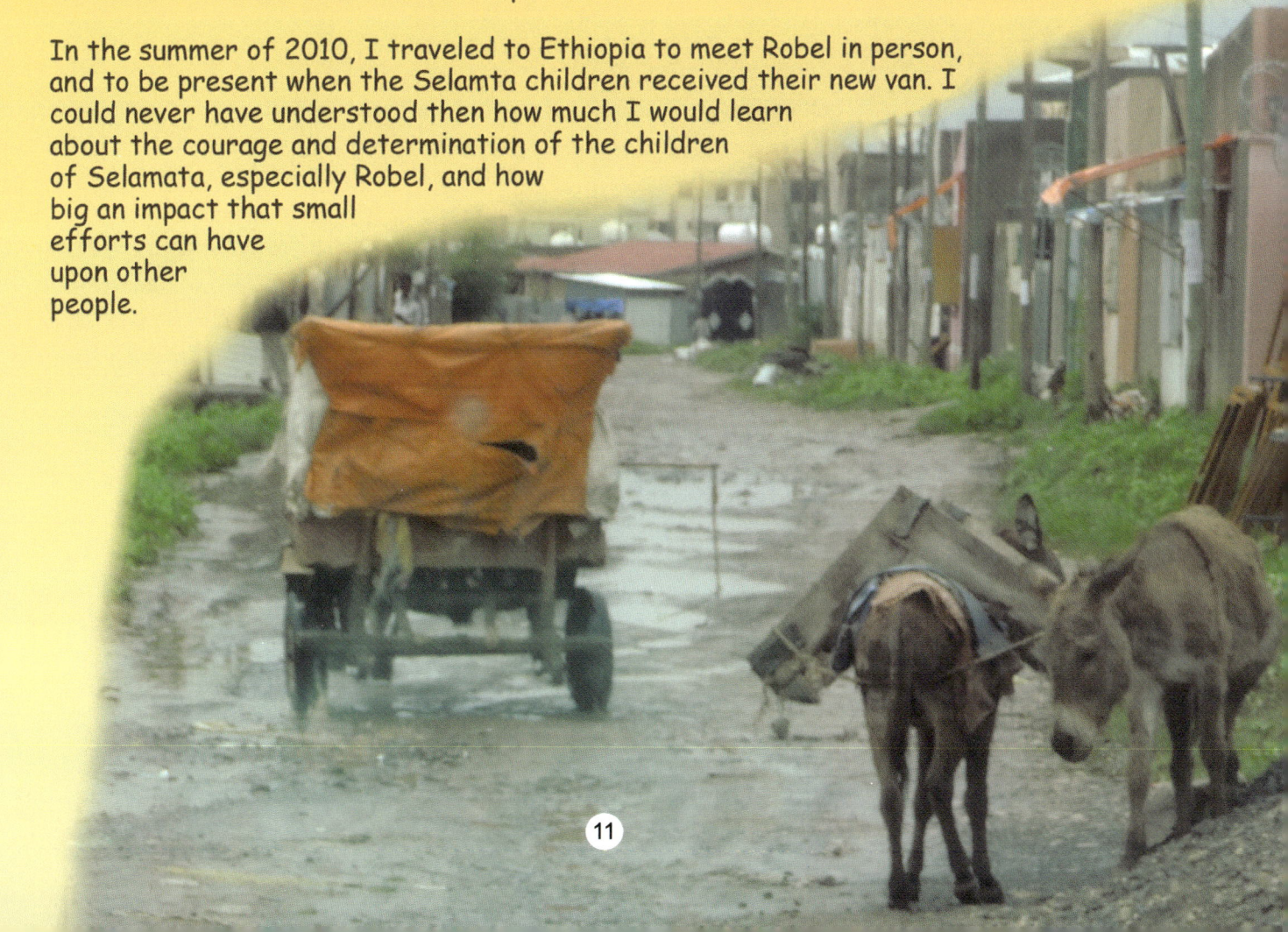

In the summer of 2010, I traveled to Ethiopia to meet Robel in person, and to be present when the Selamta children received their new van. I could never have understood then how much I would learn about the courage and determination of the children of Selamata, especially Robel, and how big an impact that small efforts can have upon other people.

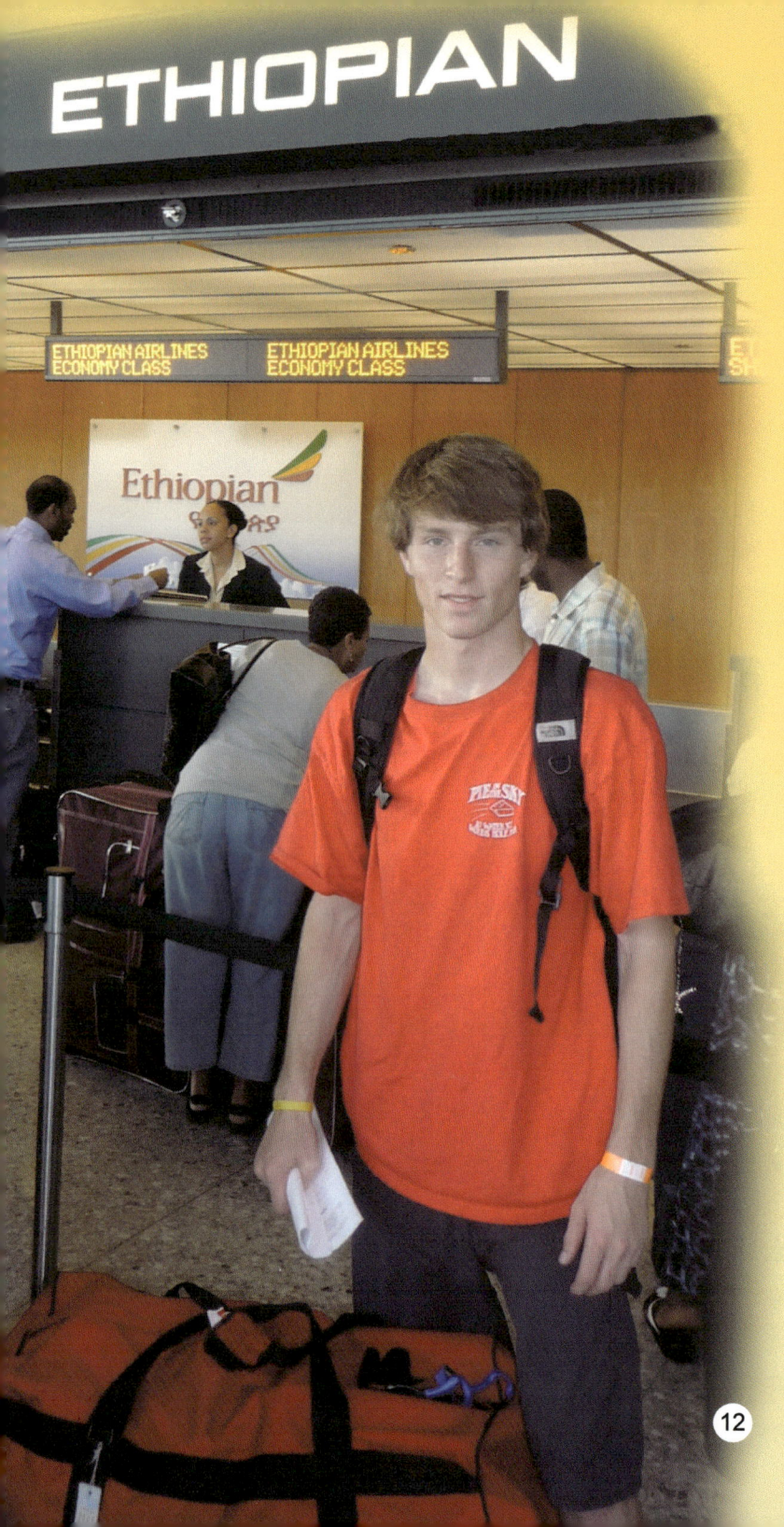

Getting to Selamta

Chris:
The day finally arrived for me to embark upon my trip to Africa. It had taken almost a year of fundraising to reach my goal of purchasing a van; the logistics of actually obtaining the vehicle had, at times, been challenging. The letters between Robel and me became even more real as I arrived at Dulles International Airport, on the outskirts of Washington, D.C., for my flight to Addis.

As I unloaded my bags from the car to check in for my flight, I had a burst of energy. I was somewhat nervous, but mostly excited to be headed over to finally meet the people of Selamta.

I had flown alone before, but nothing like the seventeen-hour flight to Rome, and then onto Addis. I plopped into my window seat, and closed my eyes. In what seemed like minutes, we landed. I had fallen asleep, and when I startled awake, I wasn't sure where I was. I didn't know whether I had slept through our refueling touchdown in Rome or not. I made my way to the door of the plane to take a peek outside, and quickly realized that the rolling hills surrounding Rome could not be the highlands of Ethiopia.

I was well rested but still anxious. I spoke with a man from Ethiopia for the remainder of the flight in an attempt to get as much information as I could. After landing in Addis, and seeing a huge sign saying, "Welcome to Ethiopia," I knew that I had finally made it! This had been more than a plane journey; this was a journey of discovery. I was ready to meet Robel, who had become such an important part of my last year.

After getting a visa and receiving my baggage, I followed a large group of people with excited faces who had just gotten off my flight as they went to seek their loved ones. It was night in Addis, and I knew that I was supposed to meet Mia Brown, the American Director of Selamta, at the airport. I nervously hoped that she remembered as well. I looked up and saw a man with a sign reading "Morse." I immediately approached him, sure that he had been sent to save me from the chaos inside the airport. The man quickly realized that I was not the "Morse" he was seeking- a man from a major corporation, coming to Addis for a business meeting. No, he wouldn't know that was a long way from the reason I was in Addis. I was a kid ready and willing to learn and embrace a new culture and community.

Thankfully, Mia identified me quickly and we left the airport to go to Bethel, a small, relatively new suburb of Addis. It was a forty minute taxi drive down an empty street, with no lights, and all I could see was Ethiopian darkness. I had no idea what I was driving by, and realized that I would wait another day to be formally introduced to Ethiopia and the families who make up the Selamta Family Project.

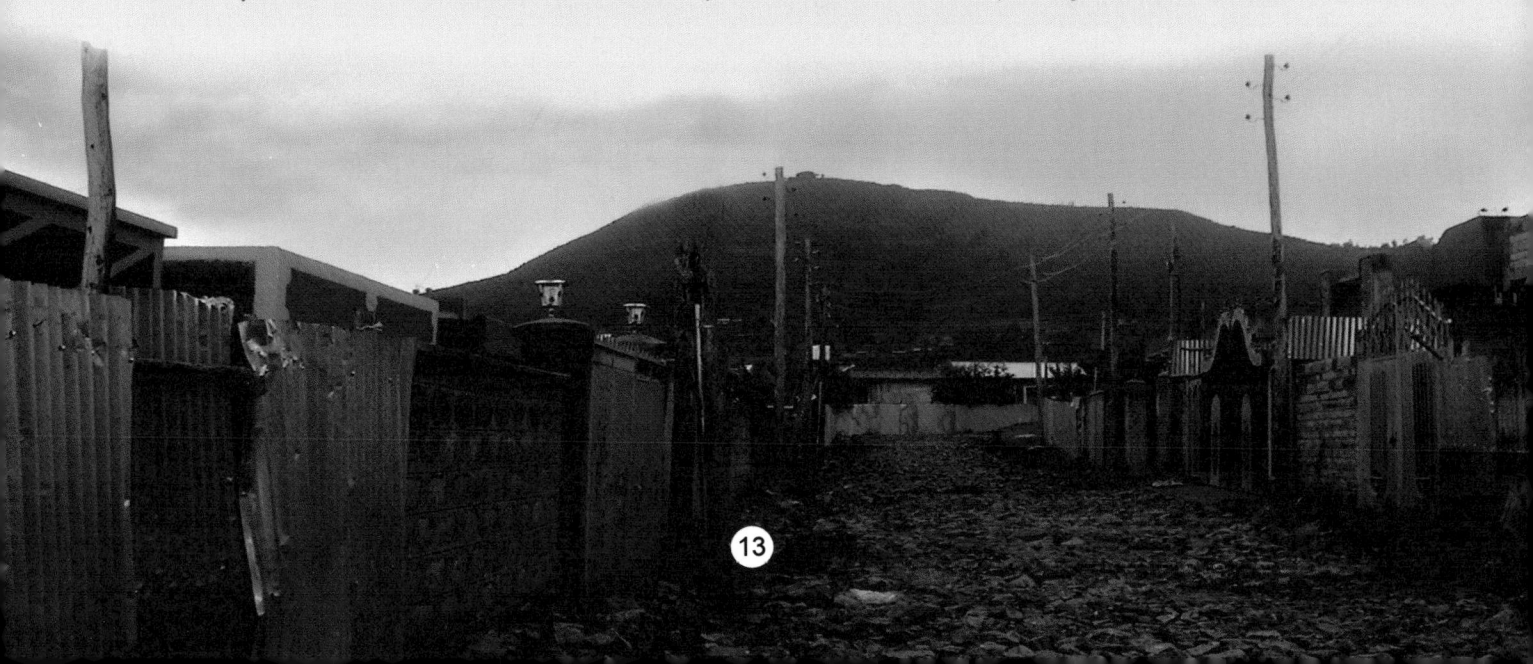

Robel:

When I was a child, I was a shepherd. I looked after cattle and sheep. My mother and my father were from two different regions; my mother from the Wolo region, and my father from the Gojam region. The town I lived in was Buja in the northern part of Ethiopia.

Our house was a hut with a roof that was thatched. It was just like other rural area houses. It was made of thatch and mud.

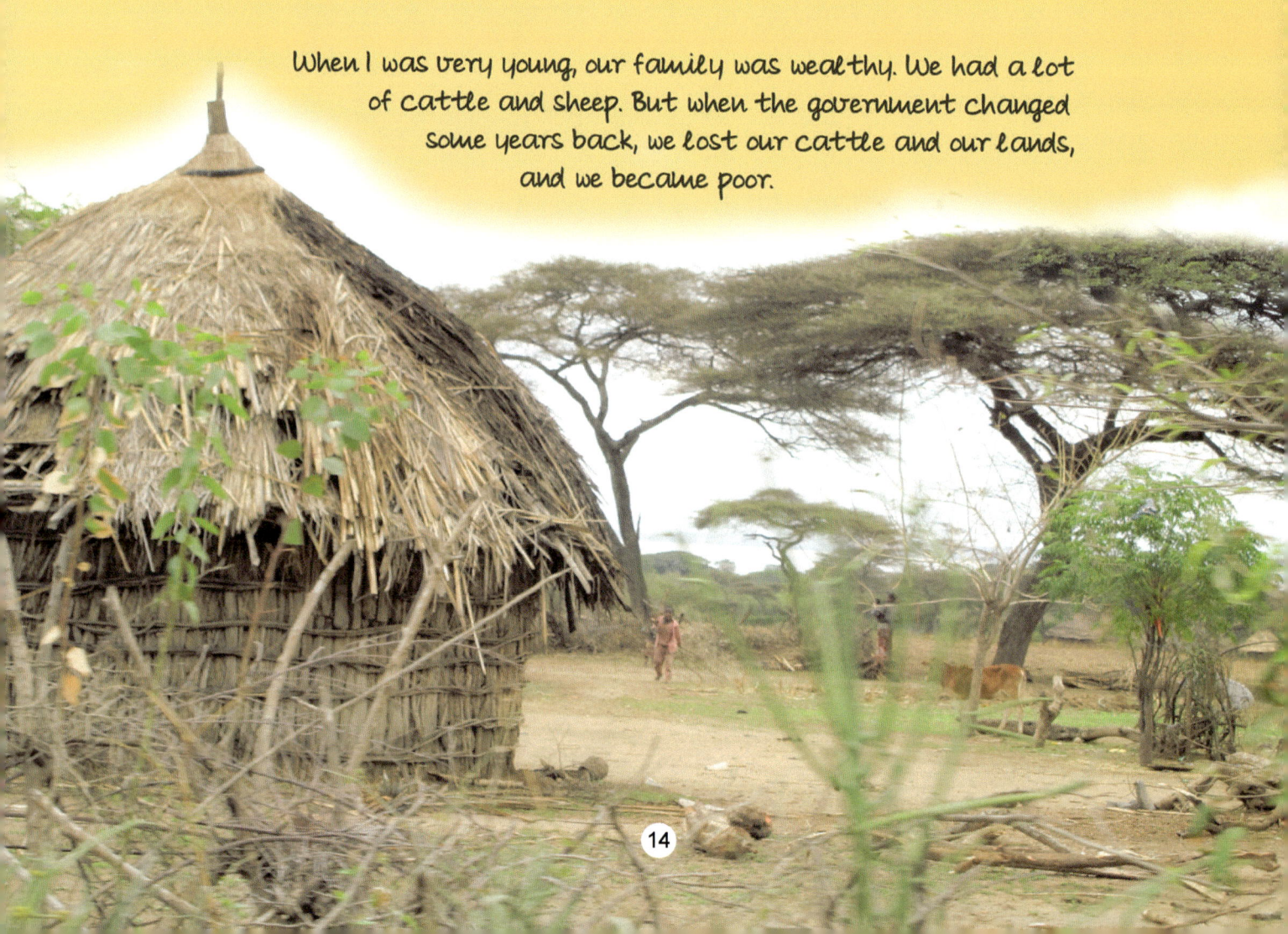

When I was very young, our family was wealthy. We had a lot of cattle and sheep. But when the government changed some years back, we lost our cattle and our lands, and we became poor.

I am sad that I don't remember my mom, but my older brother told me that I look like her. I have a vague picture of her in my mind, but truly I don't remember her. I wish that I did. She passed away when I was a child. Both my parents died, my father and my mother.

I don't know, actually, about how my father died. After we lost everything, he just got lost because he couldn't control everything in his mind. When my mother became sick, she gave us to our aunt. Then my mother passed away, and we lost all our properties.

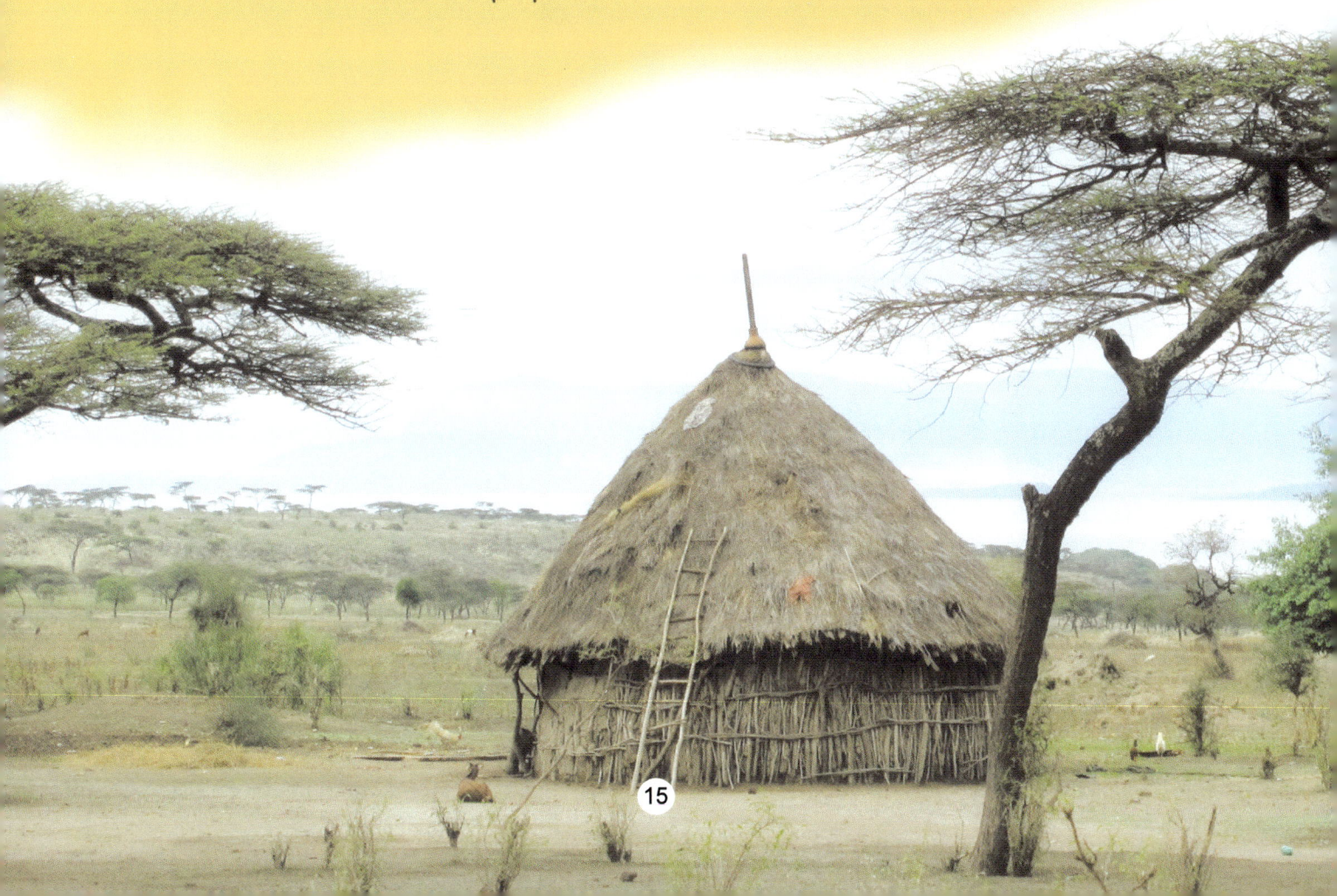

My aunt lived in Wolo so we moved from Gojam to Wolo. They are two different regions. I remember my aunt from when I first knew her. When she first met my brother and me, she was very happy. Then as time passed, things changed. She started to give us harder and harder work on her farm. We had to keep all the cattle and clean the house. After a while the work became too hard for us. She gave us food only once a day, and I wasn't allowed to go to school. I just worked on the farm. My aunt seemed to have no real interest in me.

My older brother worked on the farm for them, too. His name is Tadessa. He farmed the land and did a lot of things for them. Then, when things became too hard for him, he realized that his work on the farm was the only thing that kept him in that area. When life became even more difficult for us, my older brother finally fled the house. I remember this. I could have escaped at that time with my brother, but I thought that I needed to protect Masresha, my little brother. He was only a baby. I couldn't leave him alone, so I stayed while my older brother left.

When I was nine and Masresha was three, someone from Addis came to my area, and he talked on and on about what a good city Addis was. He told me that there was a lot of money, and it was easy to collect money on the streets. I was encouraged to come to Addis.

I was worried very much about Masresha, but I had to change my life. Because he was very young, I hoped my aunt and uncle would be kinder to him than they had been to me, and they would protect him. That's when I decided to escape.

I left Masresha, and I escaped from home early in the morning. I left and came to Addis by bus. To get the bus ticket I cried, and I begged the driver's assistant to let me on. I cried a lot, then I bowed on my knees. Finally he helped me to get onto the bus. It was one of the big busses, and it took one whole day to come to Addis. We came to the manehad (bus) station at the Mercato.

When I got there, I found street children and joined with them. When I had first thought about Addis Ababa, I expected that I would just love it. Even the name means "new flower," so I thought that there would be a lot of money and a lot of work for me, and the life here would be much better than I had in Wolo. When I came, things were not at all the same as I expected.

When I first came to Addis, I was very frightened and depressed for a month or more. I worried a lot about how my life was going to be in the future. After I made friends with some of the other street children, I started to learn about how to survive on the streets. Most of us have the same stories. We came from the countryside. Many of us came to Addis because of difficulties at home, or the death of our parents. I started to live on the streets, but at the same time I tried to search for another life. I didn't give up. I decided I could be the person in the future that I wanted to be. I was healthy, I was strong, I could work.

At first, I was living around the place called Autobistara. There are a lot of street children there, so it is very difficult to get enough leftover food from restaurants, or coins from people to survive. But in Kasanches, there are almost no street children, so it was easier to get food or to beg and get a coin. I thought life might be a little easier if I moved.

While I traveled on the road toward Kasanches, I met Teddy, the person who would soon become the closest friend I had ever had. When I talked to him I found out that we had a lot in common. He also came from the town of Bardar. We started to develop our friendship.

Teddy, he thought a lot for me. When I started smoking, he advised me not to smoke. I had a talent for singing, and he encouraged me to develop my talent. It made me want to continue when he listened to me and appreciated my music. He helped me a lot, and he was a good friend to me.

After we had lived on the streets for four years, Teddy and I knew that we needed to make a change in our lives. We had heard that other children had joined organizations that had provided food and shelter. Teddy had the idea that we should find an organization like this, and he shared his idea with me.

I asked him how we would find an organization that would take us, since I had no idea. There seemed to be many organizations, and most of them were for people who were HIV positive or who had AIDS, which we didn't. It was very confusing. He said, "Let's just go and ask the people who are in the sub-city offices for help."

The sub-cities are sections of Addis. We went to see the sub-city administrator, and we asked him to help us. He wrote a letter to the Social Affairs Office.

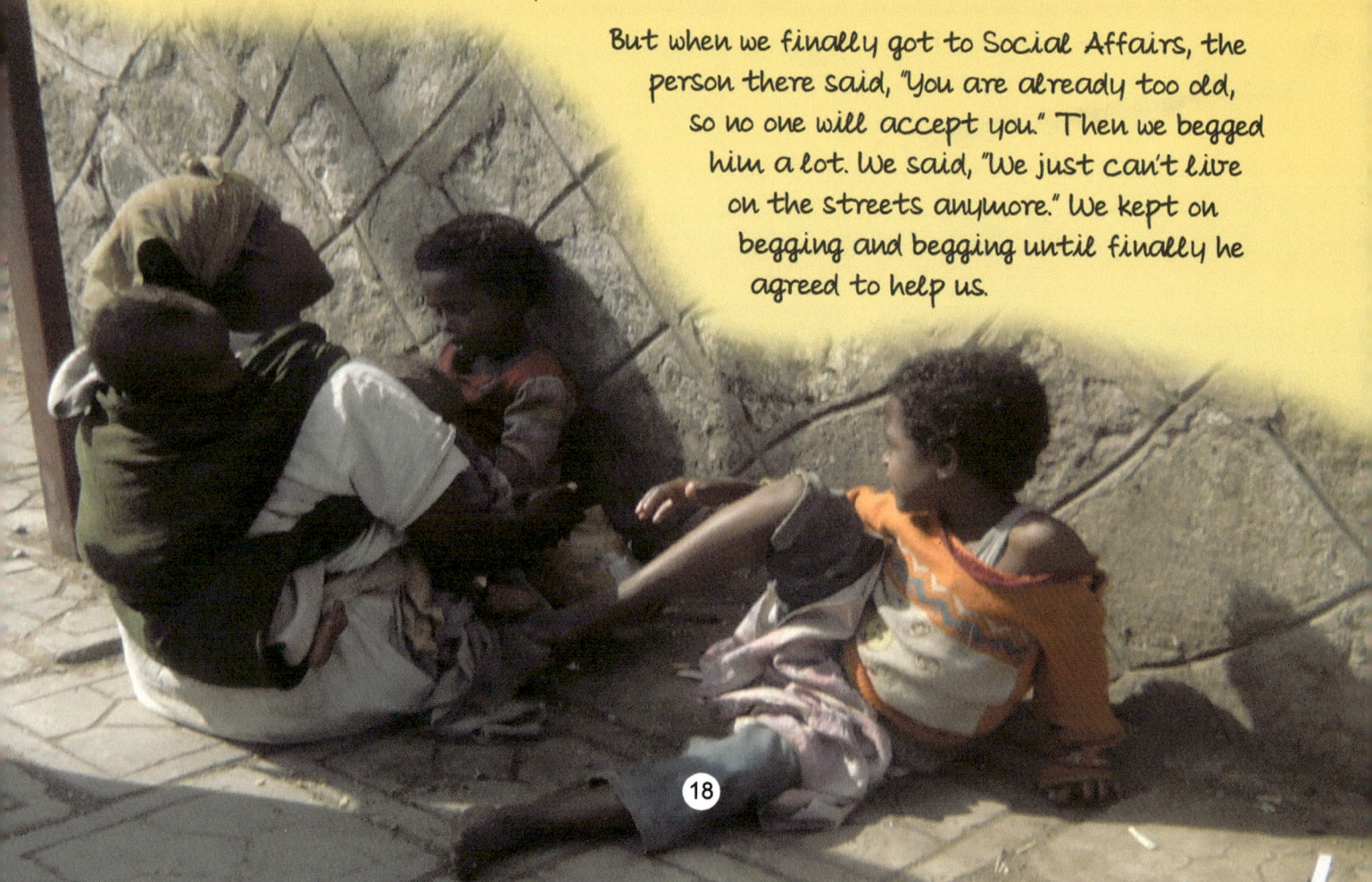

But when we finally got to Social Affairs, the person there said, "You are already too old, so no one will accept you." Then we begged him a lot. We said, "We just can't live on the streets anymore." We kept on begging and begging until finally he agreed to help us.

At last, the administrator sent us to an organization that he thought could take us in. We were very excited that we might finally have a new home. But when we got there, they told us that we needed to have someone who would account for us; a relative or family member. The man said that he was not allowed to let us in without this verification. Neither of us had any parents or family members to verify us. He finally said, "We will not accept you. It's very full."

We were very sad and discouraged, so we went back to the Social Affairs Office. Especially after the first organization had refused us, we would go to the Social Affairs Office every week on Friday to ask them to find us a better organization.

We asked them again and again for three reasons. The first was that we wanted a better life than we had as street children. The second was that we wanted to have a chance to have clean, healthy food so we would feel better. The third was that we hoped to have an education so we could do something valuable with our lives.

Then the man there told us about the Selamta Family Project. At first we worried that it was a foundation or organization just for HIV carriers, but we found out that was not true. The Social Affairs Officer told the people at Selamta that there were two boys who really wanted to join their organization. Finally, he just let me talk directly with the person at Selamta. I was very surprised when the person on the phone said, "Wait for us in the place where you sleep with your papers. We will come there to pick you up."

Just as they had promised, they came around to get us right where we were living, and brought us to Selamta. It took one whole year from when we first went to the Social Affairs Office until the time we came to Selamta. On August 18th, 2008 we became part of the Selamta Family Project and had a new family. On that day our lives were changed forever.

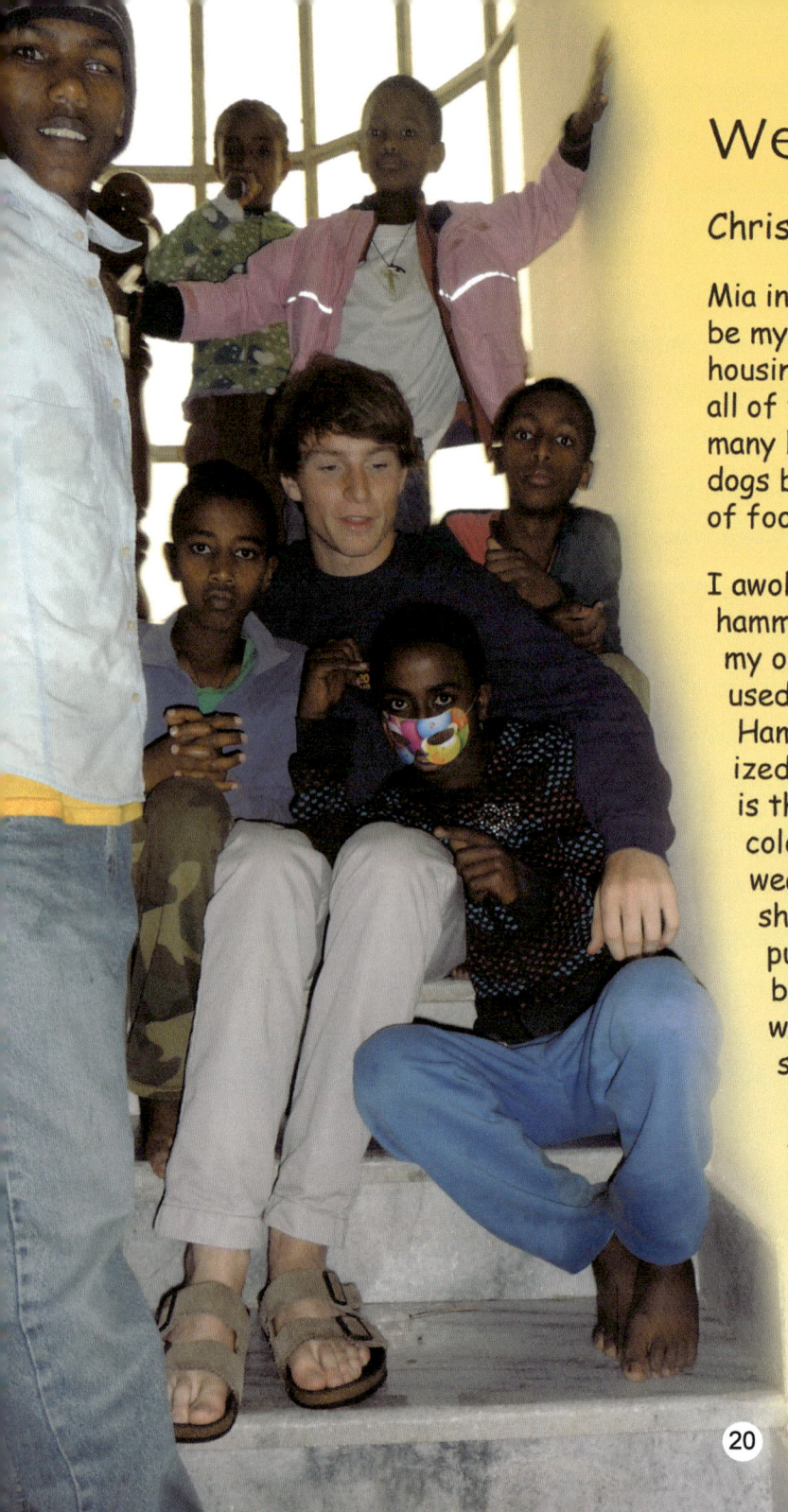

Welcome to the Family

Chris:

Mia introduced me to the "Inn," which would be my home while I was at Selamta. My housing was located within a mile from where all of the families of Selamta live. After many hours of listening to neighborhood dogs barking, yelping, and fighting for scraps of food, I finally fell asleep.

I awoke on my first day in Ethiopia to a loud hammering noise that sounded like it was in my own room. This startled me since I am used to the peace and quiet of the New Hampshire countryside, but I quickly realized that this noise and abundant activity is the norm in Ethiopia. I was jetlagged, cold, and confused… but awake. I was wearing the same sweatpants and sweatshirt that I hardly remembered having put on in my exhaused state the night before. I was glad for the extra warmth since this was the cold and rainy season in Ethiopia. The Ethiopian highlands are not the Sahara desert! Addis, on its geographically raised platform, stands several thousand feet above sea level, making the climate much colder than I had anticipated for Africa.

As I meandered down from the top floor of the office building, there were over fifty young kids waiting in the Selamta common room for a woman who was going to teach them "life skills." These life skills included learning things like CPR, knitting, human anatomy, constructing simple tools, and generally furthering their fund of useful knowledge.

I was happy to see that Selamta was preparing the kids for the real world with life skills. As I looked into that room, I was overwhelmed with the amount of excitement, and the smiles on the children's faces. While they waited, the kids were occupying themselves by coloring, talking, dancing and watching a video on fast-forward.

I would soon realize how much Selamta children enjoyed playing videos on fast-forward. Perhaps, I thought, it was because these children try to see and learn everything at top speed, or perhaps it was just that they didn't understand the language, so they were more intrigued by the movie's actions.

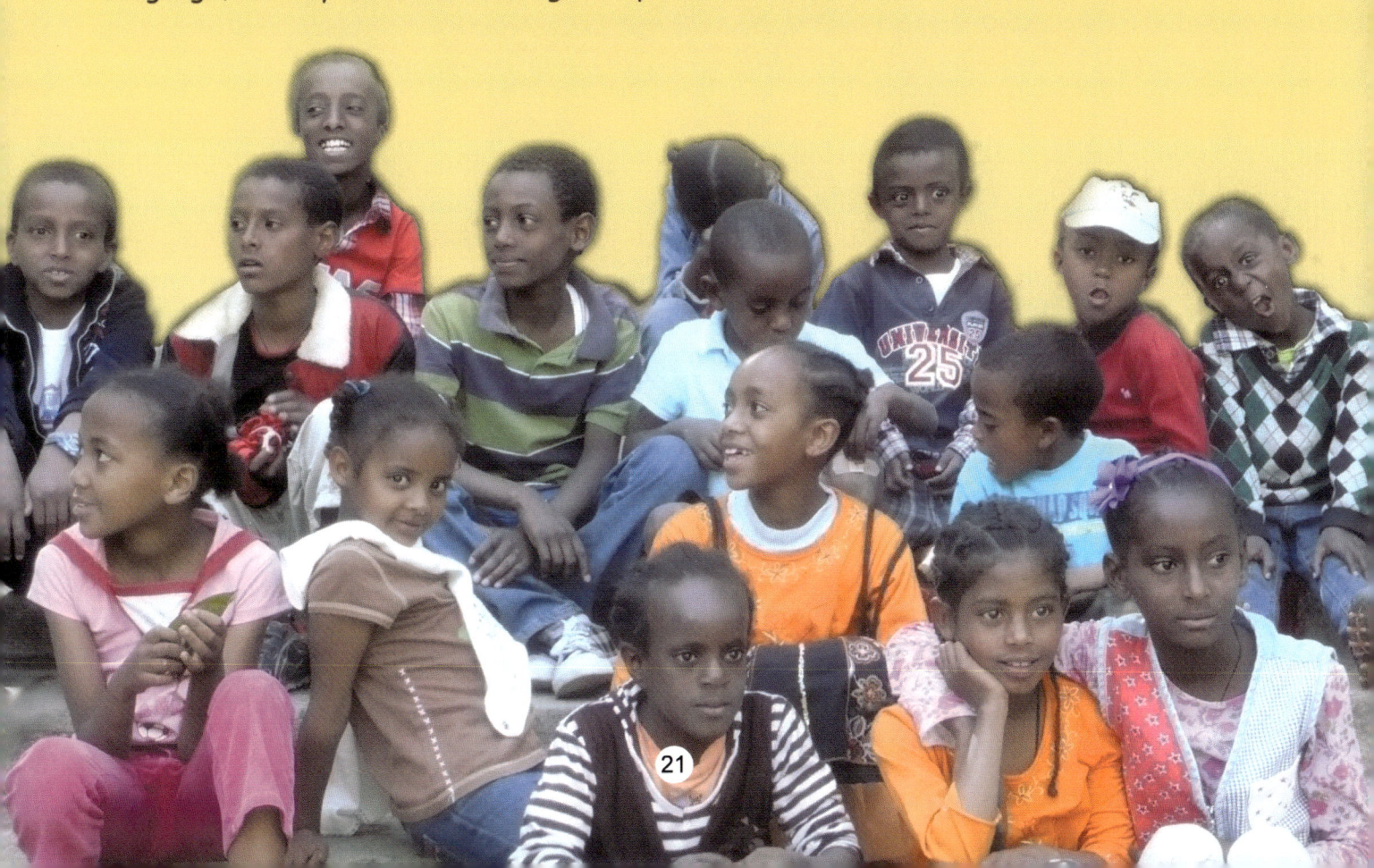

22

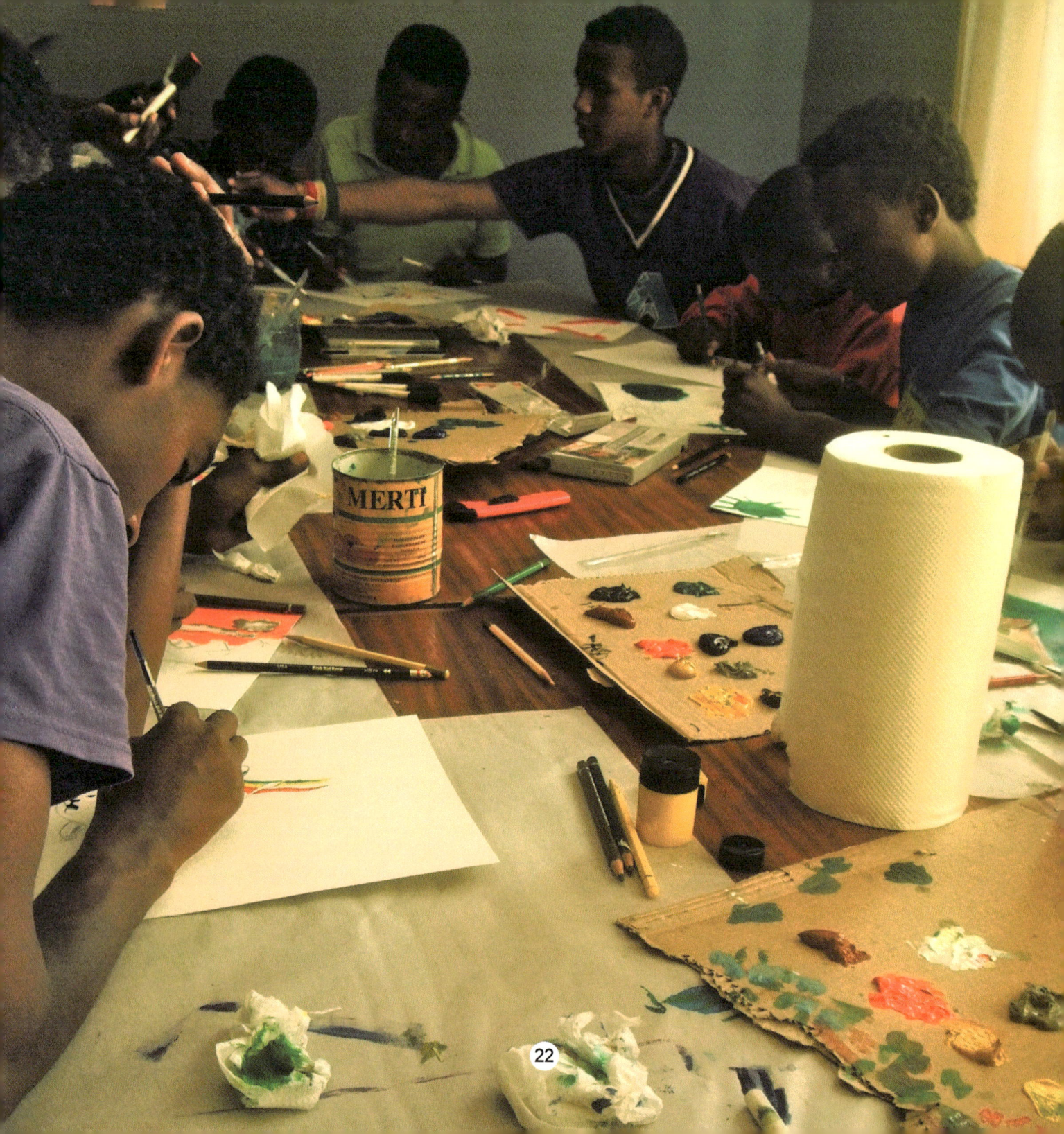

When the kids looked up from their activities and saw me enter the room, there was a hush as they peered up at this stranger. The boys and several outgoing older girls came to introduce themselves to me. They spoke their native Amharic and some broken English. Considering many of these kids had come from life on the streets and had received little to no formal education before getting to Selamta, it was surprising how many spoke at least some English. Mostly, though, they just smiled at me or tried to draw a picture for me with their age, name and grade level as a way of introduction.

I stood and watched the kids, enchanted by their cute faces, big smiles and strange language. After several hours, the kids scattered back to their family homes for lunch.

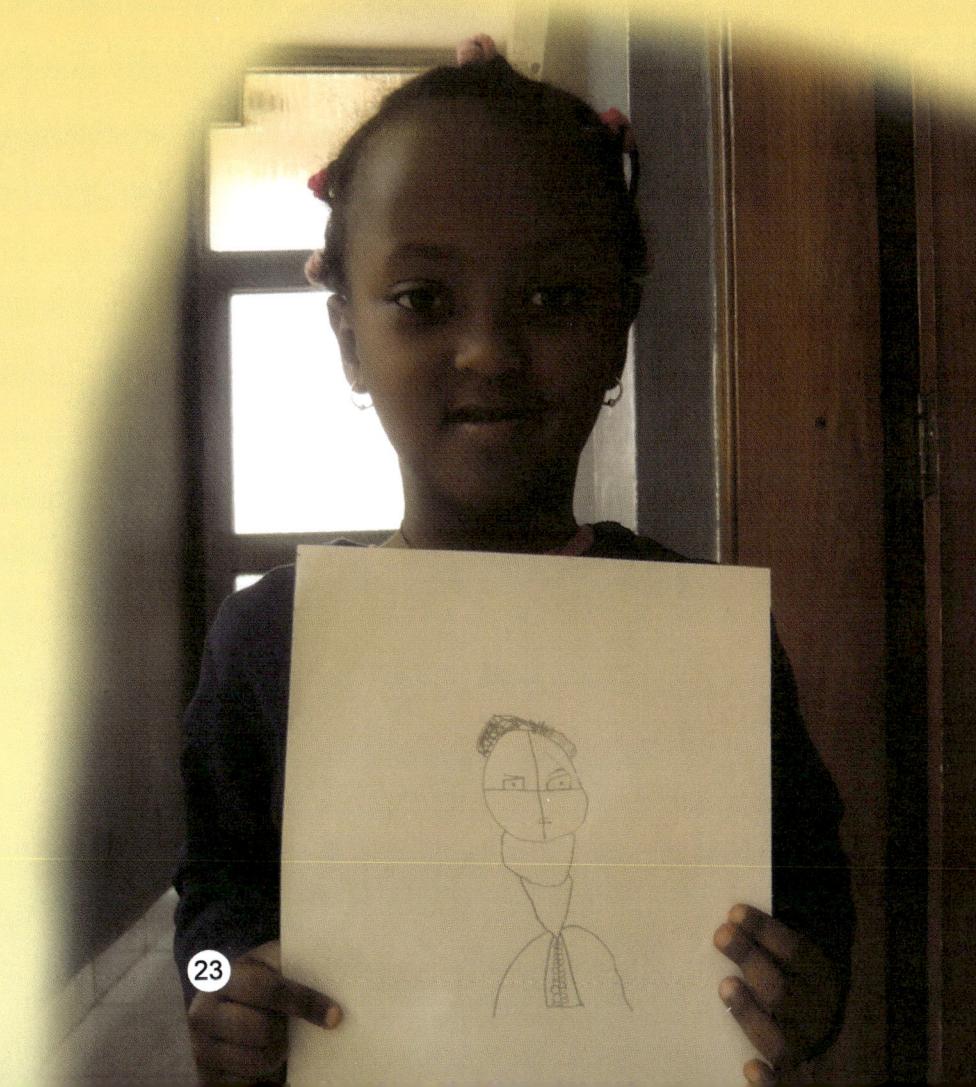

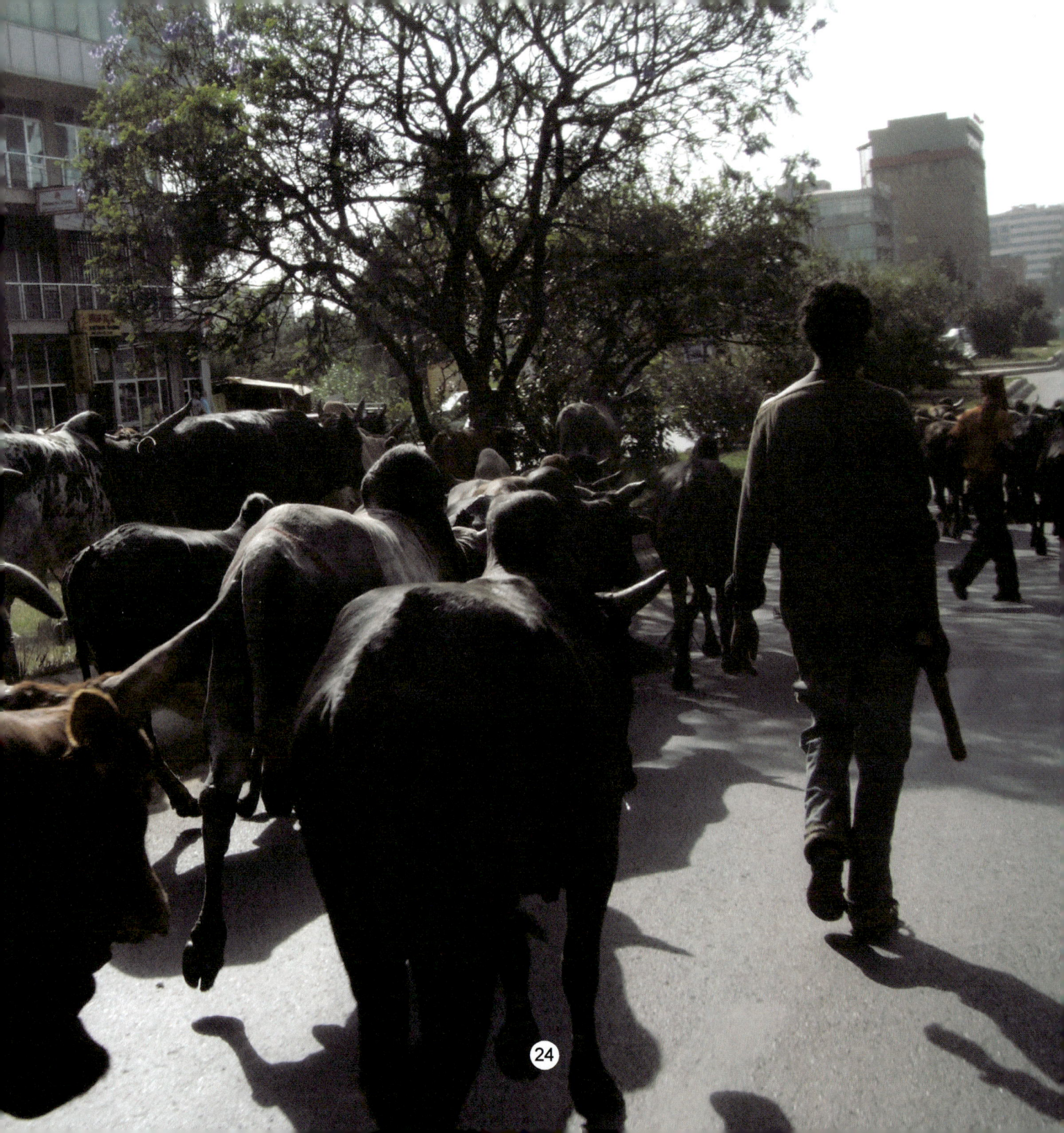

After my own lunch, I had my first "buna" time. This is the traditional Ethiopian coffee ceremony that happens every day following lunch. It involves hand grinding the coffee, roasting it over a small fire, brewing it and serving it in its strongest form. The expectation is that you drink three cups. As I tasted my first espresso shot of coffee, I was pretty sure that I would be awake for the rest of the day!

I then walked into the town of Bethel and saw the streets lined with people carrying countless household and personal items. Dogs, goats, and horses roamed aimlessly through these streets. This was an opening to an entirely new world.

The new van was a surprise for all the kids, and we were having a party the next day to make the announcement. Mia and I hopped into a taxi to head into downtown Addis to get supplies for the celebration.

A constant stream of people, cars, and animals moves through the streets of Addis. Every street is alive with people figuring out how they can sell merchandise or use their skills to make a few Birr, in a country where the average person lives off $2 a day. Stores sell goods through windows. Kids clean shoes, or carry massive bags filled with literally anything. Women with babies and disabled people asking for change mesh into the countless people lining the streets. I was stunned at the vast number of cars traveling haphazardly down the crowded streets.

We stopped at Kaldi's Coffee shop where I had my first encounter with street children. As I approached the coffee shop door, two street children begged me for money and food. I wasn't used to people begging to strangers, much less children begging on the streets. Without hesitation,

26

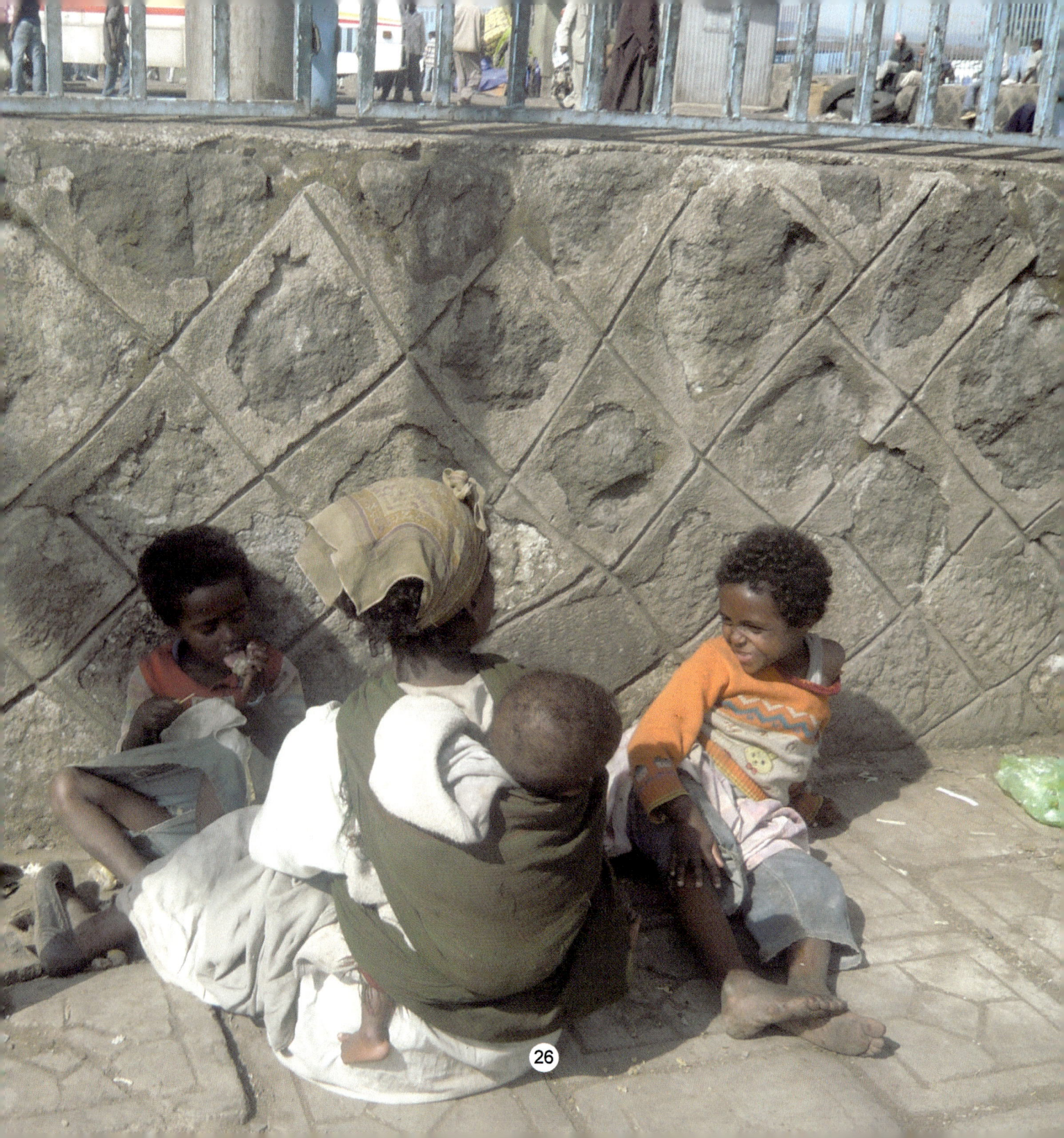

I gave them 10 Birr ($1 is 17 Birr) and then headed into get some food. Seeing their faces peering through the window made me feel so guilty that I couldn't eat, so I left and gave the children the food. It made me so sad to see these two young kids on the streets- the first two of thousands that I would see in Ethiopia.

After getting party supplies and finally making our way back to Selamta, we were exhausted. Going several miles using public transportation is expensive and time consuming. I realized how helpful the van would be in solving both of these problems. We had a quick dinner and then went to bed.

I couldn't sleep as I kept thinking about the street children I had seen. I didn't have any way to know then of the real devistation that life on the steets entails. It was only later as I heard some of the horrific stories from Robel as we traveled some of the paths of his earlier life did I begin to understand the implications of life on the streets. I was, however, acutely aware of how much the lives of Selamta's children had been changed as a result of the Selamta Family Project.

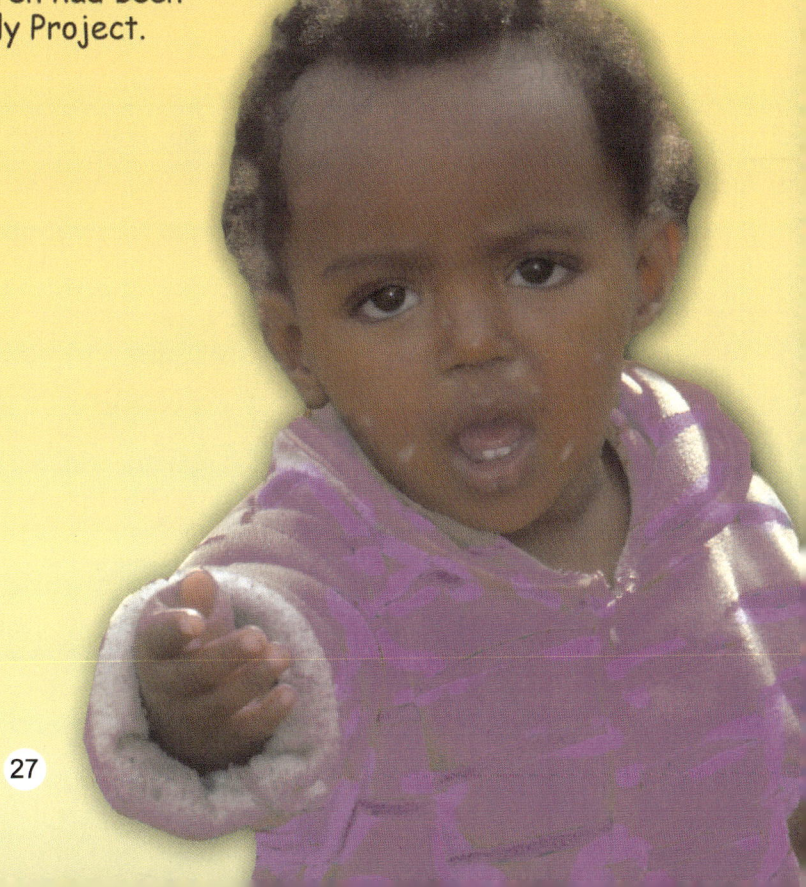

The Van

Chris:
Again I awoke to loud hammering, and realized that the noises were coming from an adjacent building. I was excited about the scheduled party and to finally meet my friend, Robel. I hoped that he would be as excited to meet me as I was to meet him. Esmael, a twenty-five year old native Ethiopian, who had been friend to the Selamta project for years, came to pick us up in the new van.

It was bright white, had three rows of seats, and would blend in nicely with the other countless vehicles on those crazy Ethiopian roads. The van is equipped to transport people over both paved and unpaved roads, making it particularly useful to Selamta. As Mia and I were making the final preparations prior to presenting the van to the community, Esmael drove Mia and me back into Addis to secure more party supplies.

After some time driving on the roads of Addis with animals, people and other vehicles moving rapidly in every direction in front of us, I looked out the van window, I saw a big "S" marking the five-star Sheraton Hotel. This hotel, with its lavish exterior stood in sharp contrast to the traditional housing, built from eucalyptus trees and tin scraps held together with mud cement. The contrasting wealth and poverty was remarkable. As the sky began its downpour, the countless street children scattered for cover in a vain attempt to stay dry. Watching those children empty out of their streets in search of shelter, I realized that for them, any shelter was merely temporary.

We arrived back at Selamta and earnestly began party preparations. We blew up balloons, put out party hats, and distributed bowls full of sweets and drinks. I was reminded that following the party, every single bottle had to be returned, for in Ethiopia the bottle is worth more than the drink.

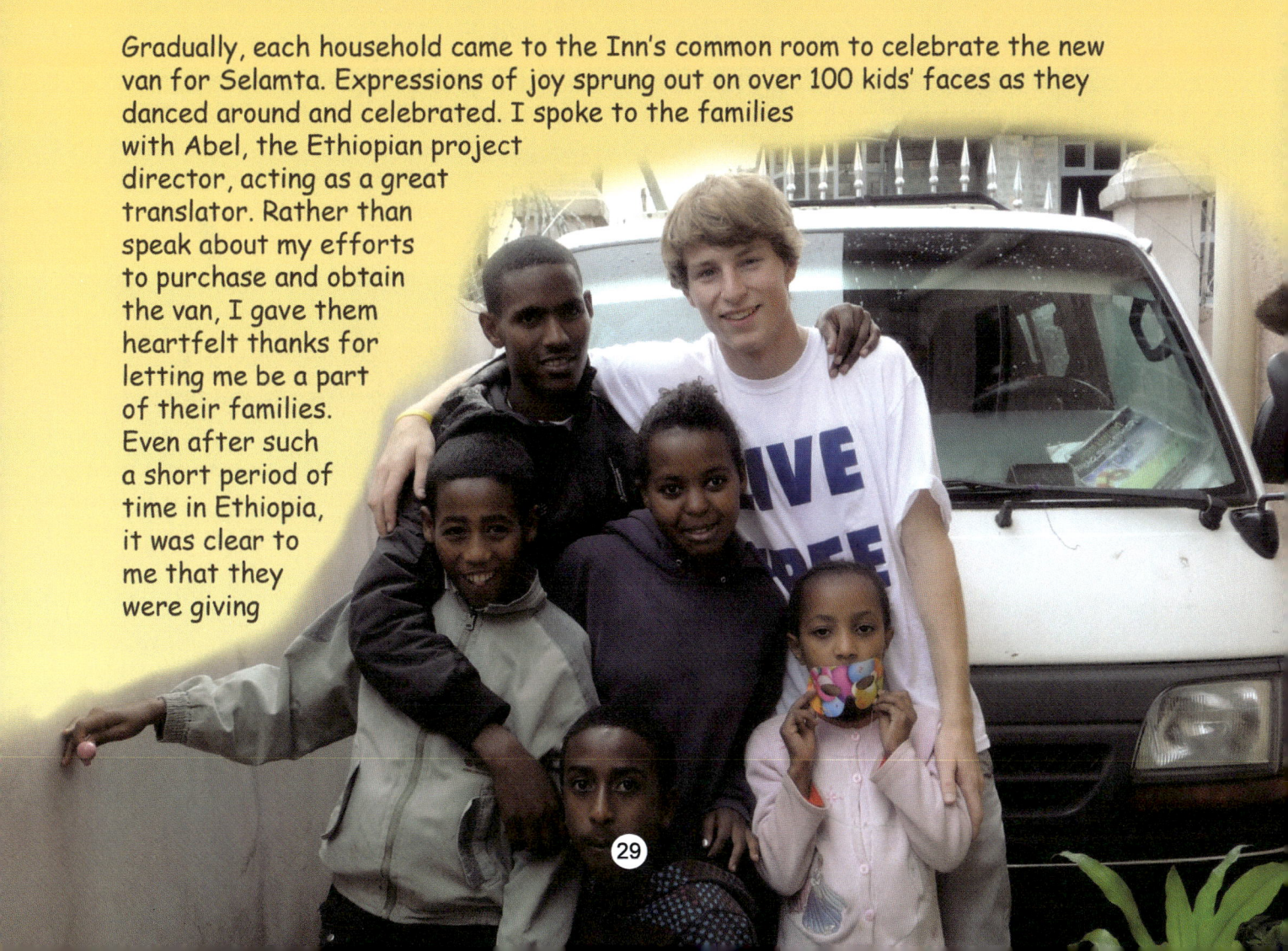

Gradually, each household came to the Inn's common room to celebrate the new van for Selamta. Expressions of joy sprung out on over 100 kids' faces as they danced around and celebrated. I spoke to the families with Abel, the Ethiopian project director, acting as a great translator. Rather than speak about my efforts to purchase and obtain the van, I gave them heartfelt thanks for letting me be a part of their families. Even after such a short period of time in Ethiopia, it was clear to me that they were giving more to me than they realized, and I wanted to hug each child and thank them. As the kids started to file out to return to their homes, and the older kids helped with the clean up, I was approached by a tall, slender Ethiopian boy who I recognized must be Robel.

Finally, I got to meet my friend. At first he appeared nervous and shy, speaking each English word hesitantly. Robel is my age, yet he is much shorter than my six-foot frame. As we spoke, I gradually learned more and more about his past life. I knew immediately that this was the beginning of a life-long friendship.

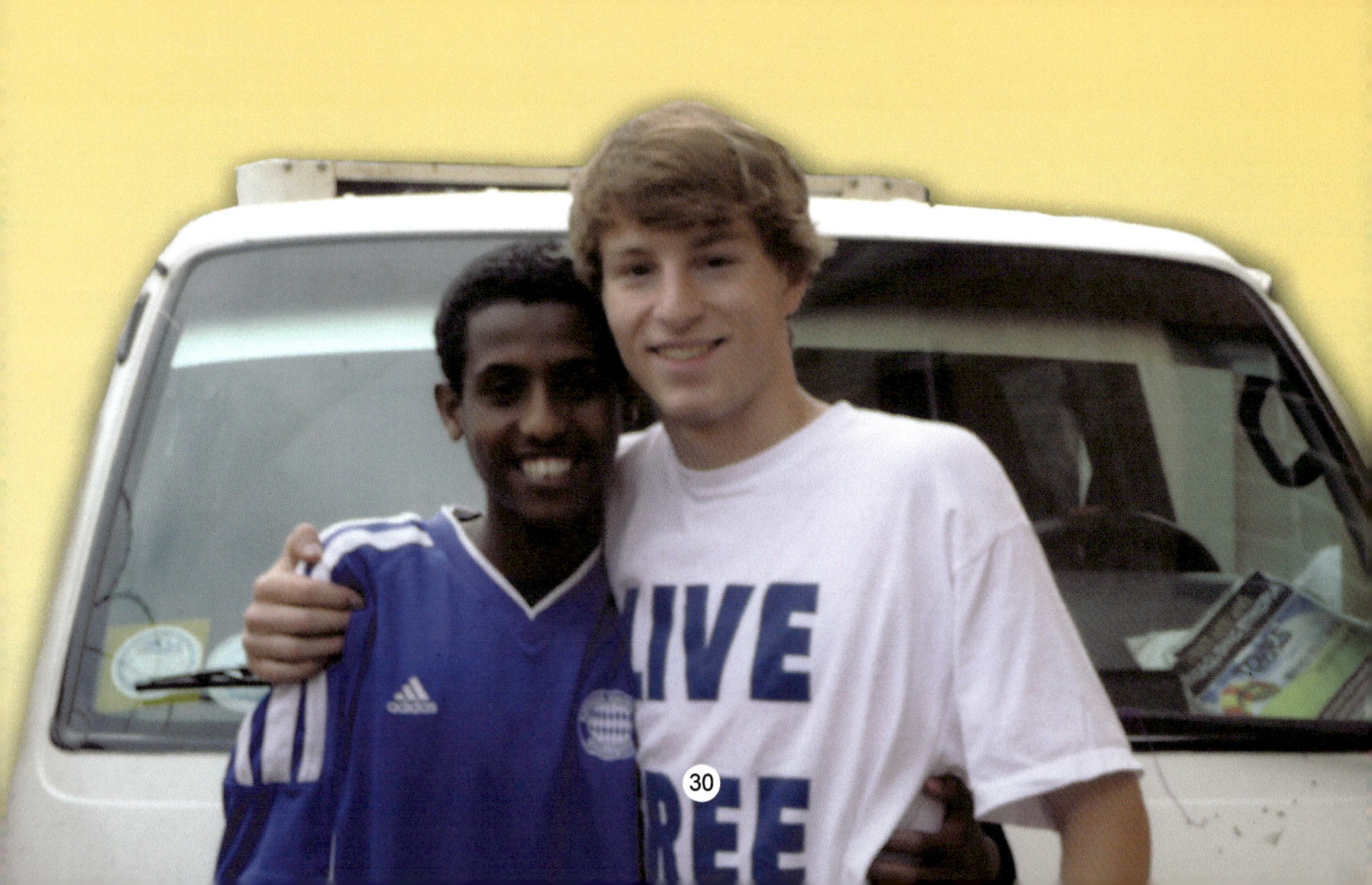

Robel:

Chris is a very lovable guy. I was so happy to meet him. It was a little bit difficult for me to communicate with him because I am not so good at speaking English. I understood him when he spoke, but it was sometimes difficult for me to explain things. I used words that I knew in English, and he usually understood me. He has done so much for all of us at Selamta, and he has helped me out in many ways. He has worked very hard for us. I was very happy to meet Chris finally.

I clapped a lot and I shouted when I heard that Chris got us the van. I was shocked! I was very happy that he raised the money for the van because a car is so very necessary for us. We always asked to have a car for Selamta because if something bad happens here in the nighttime, there is no way to take kids to the hospital. It's really a necessary thing. I shouted a lot with happiness!

The thing is, life has become very difficult here in Ethiopia because the exchange rate is increasing so quickly. Everything becomes so expensive. Rather than buying things around here in Bethel, it is better to buy from the Merkato, or a store near the source. The car is necessary to go and buy these things. It's really important to us.

The Circus

Chris:

I prepared to go to the "Circus" with a large group of Selamta children. In America, a circus would have elephants, horses, clowns, trapeze gymnasts, as well as a vast array of what parents call "junk food." I had a suspicion that this Ethiopian circus would be quite different. The circus had been rented specifically for the Selamta children to enjoy. The circus was in a few suburbs over from where the houses were located. We started our twenty minute walk to the circus - a pack of African children and one white American, me.

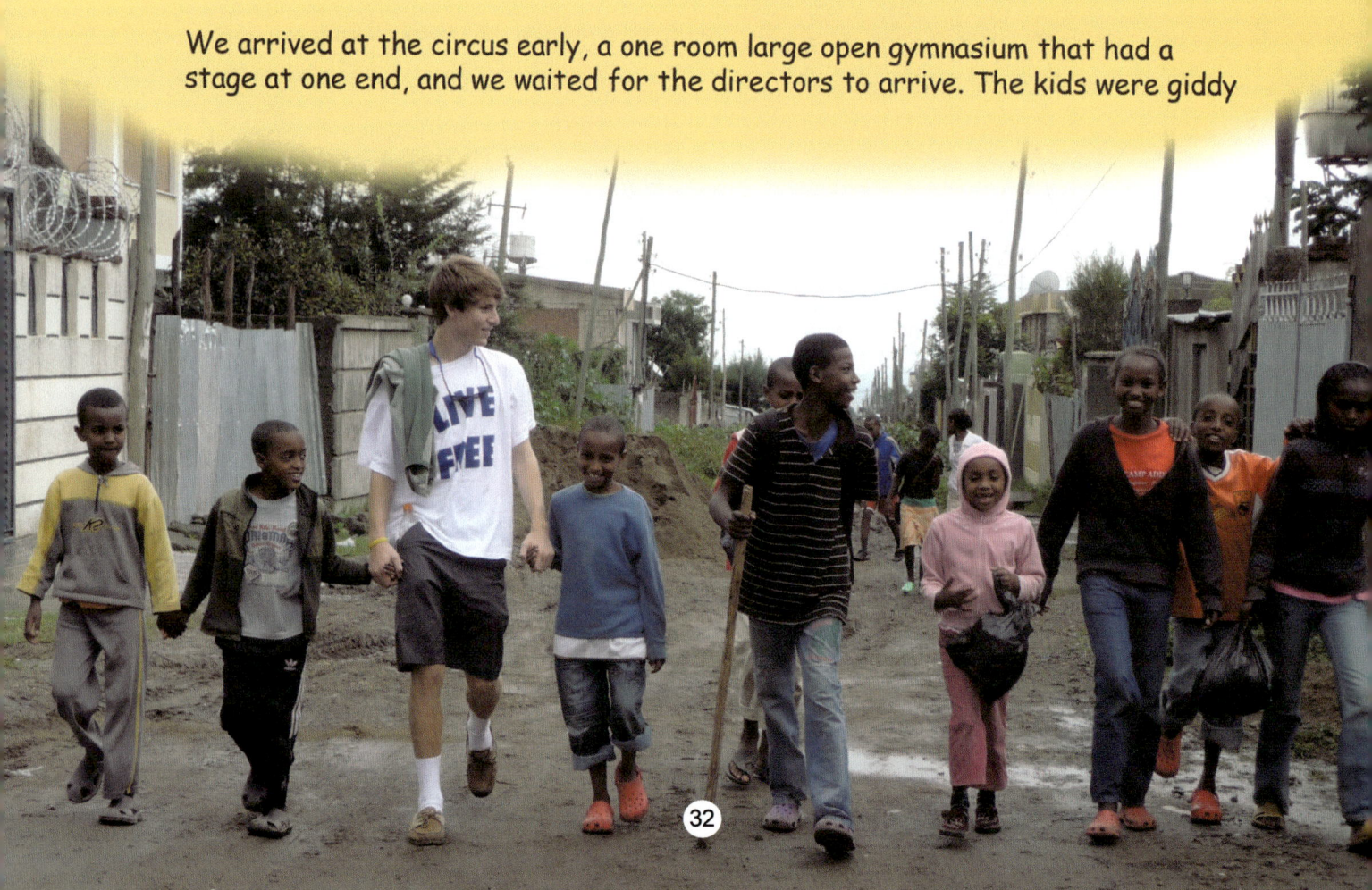

We arrived at the circus early, a one room large open gymnasium that had a stage at one end, and we waited for the directors to arrive. The kids were giddy with excitement knowing that the activities would soon begin. There were many faces, each of which held a smile.

Once the directors arrived with a few co-workers, the students lined up in single file going from the front with the stage to the back of the open gym. Each student warmed up in preparation for various physical activities. I realized that this Ethiopian circus was more like an American gymnastics program, and that the real circus participants were actually the Selamta children themselves.

One end of the gym was for juggling, hacky sac and other yo-yo like games. Further beyond this was an area for dancing. The Selamta children began running around doing splits, cartwheels, and handstands, impressing me with their speed and agility. Children wanted me to participate with them, but their skills were much better than mine. We were there for over three hours with few breaks and had lots of fun. After a brief closing talk by the director, the kids dispersed to the streets and headed back to Selamta.

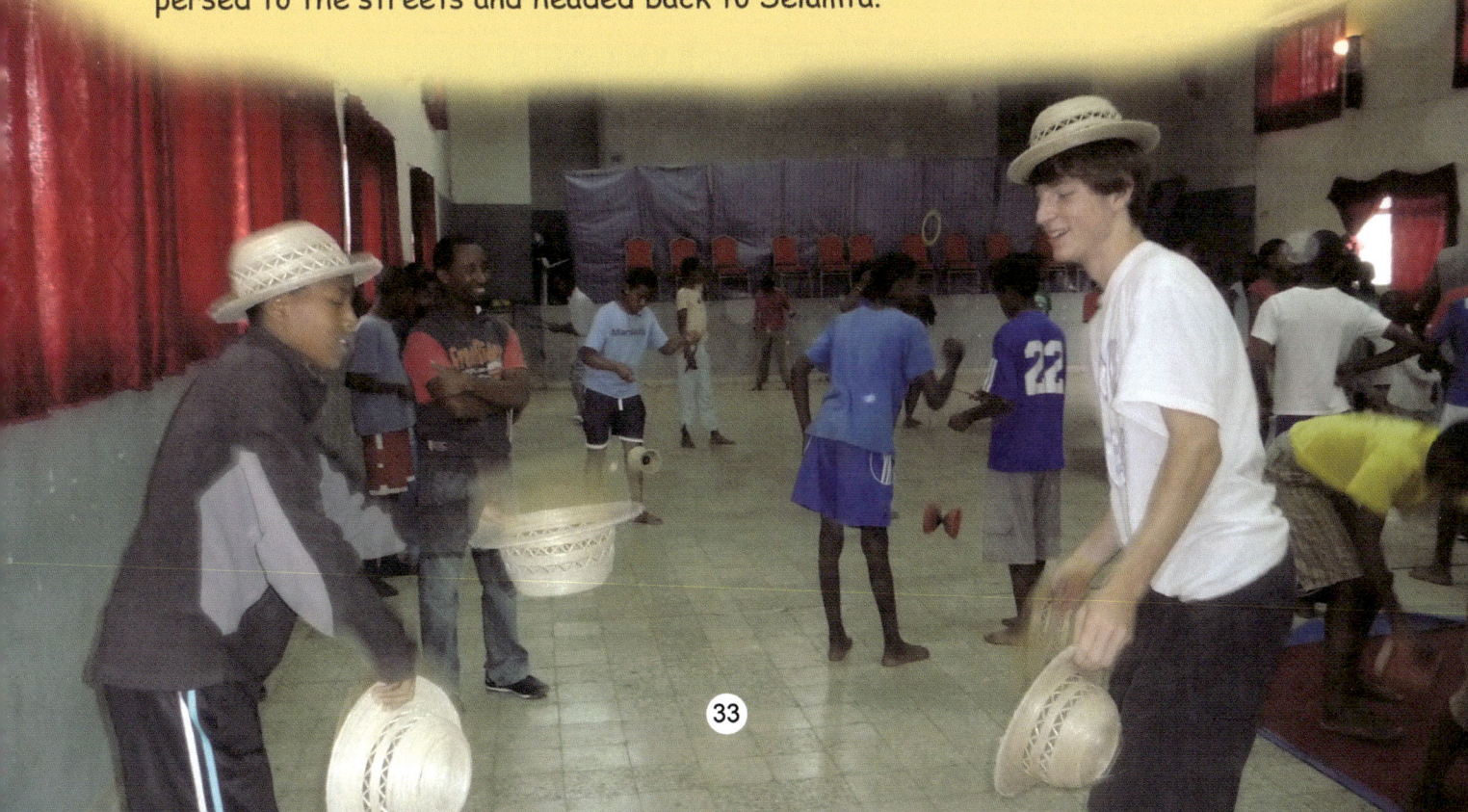

To the Hospital

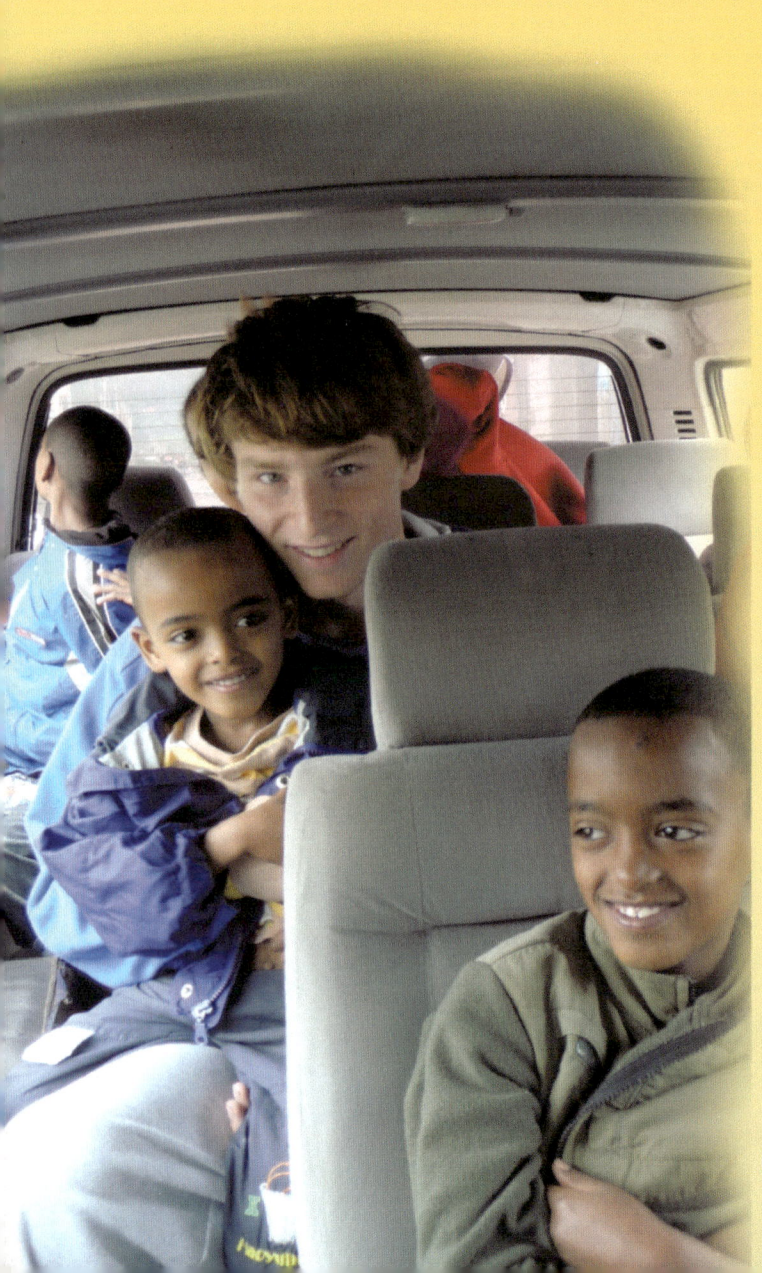

Chris

Going to the hospital in an emergency is a frightening experience for most kids. One of the most significant uses for the new van is as an emergency vehicle when kids need medical help. We had the chance to take one Selamta family to the hospital in Bethel so they could see it before there was an emergency situation. We loaded the kids into the van, and headed off to Bethel Hospital. Most of the children had never been in a car before, but here were ten kids piled into the van.

As we grew nearer to the hospital, we stopped at a small shop selling Mirindas on the side of the road. Mirindas are like American soft drinks, and the kids love them, so there were many smiles.

Giving the kids a chance to see the hospital in a circumstance that was fun will reduce fear and stress when a real emergency does occur.

35

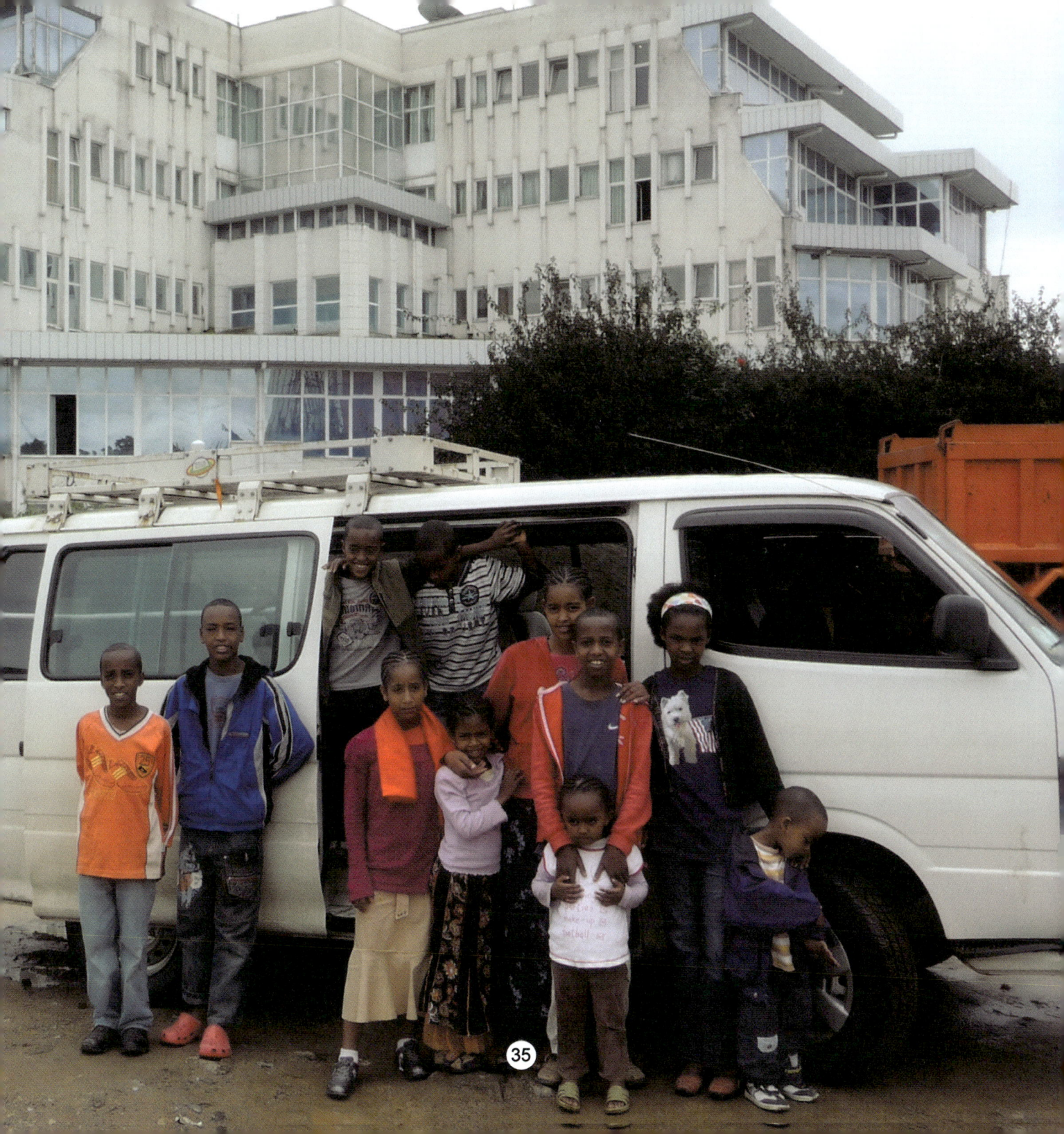

Futball (Soccer)

Chris:

A small group of children escorted Mia and me back to the "Inn." We ate lunch, and then Robel and Nati came to get me to play soccer. They presented me with a pair of cleats. I was glad to have a pair of cleats, even though they were four sizes too small. In a country like Ethiopia, complaining about something, like shoes being too small, isn't done. We ran from family unit to family unit, in order to gather enough players for two teams.

We headed towards the outskirts of Addis onto the hillside with open fields surrounded by grazing cattle and donkeys. The soccer field was muddy, wet, slippery, and sparsely laden with rocks and sticks—quite a contrast to the astro-turf soccer field where American teams play. I quickly learned that they could clearly play soccer, with refined and superior skills to mine. Many local people stopped to watch our game, and were mesmerized by the fact that a "ferengi" (foreigner) was out in the middle of a wet soccer field in a remote suburb of Addis.

Robel:

For me, futball is my entertainment. Sometimes I play futball with the children. I would not play futball for a living, but I do like to play sometimes for fun.

I think futball helps the Selamta kids to entertain themselves, but in our country's context, I don't think futball is a way out, for a living, for a future. But for entertainment, it's nice. When I play futball with the children, I teach them some skills that I have. I am careful not to say bad words with them, or things like that. I play like a child. When I play with older boys or men, I feel like a man.

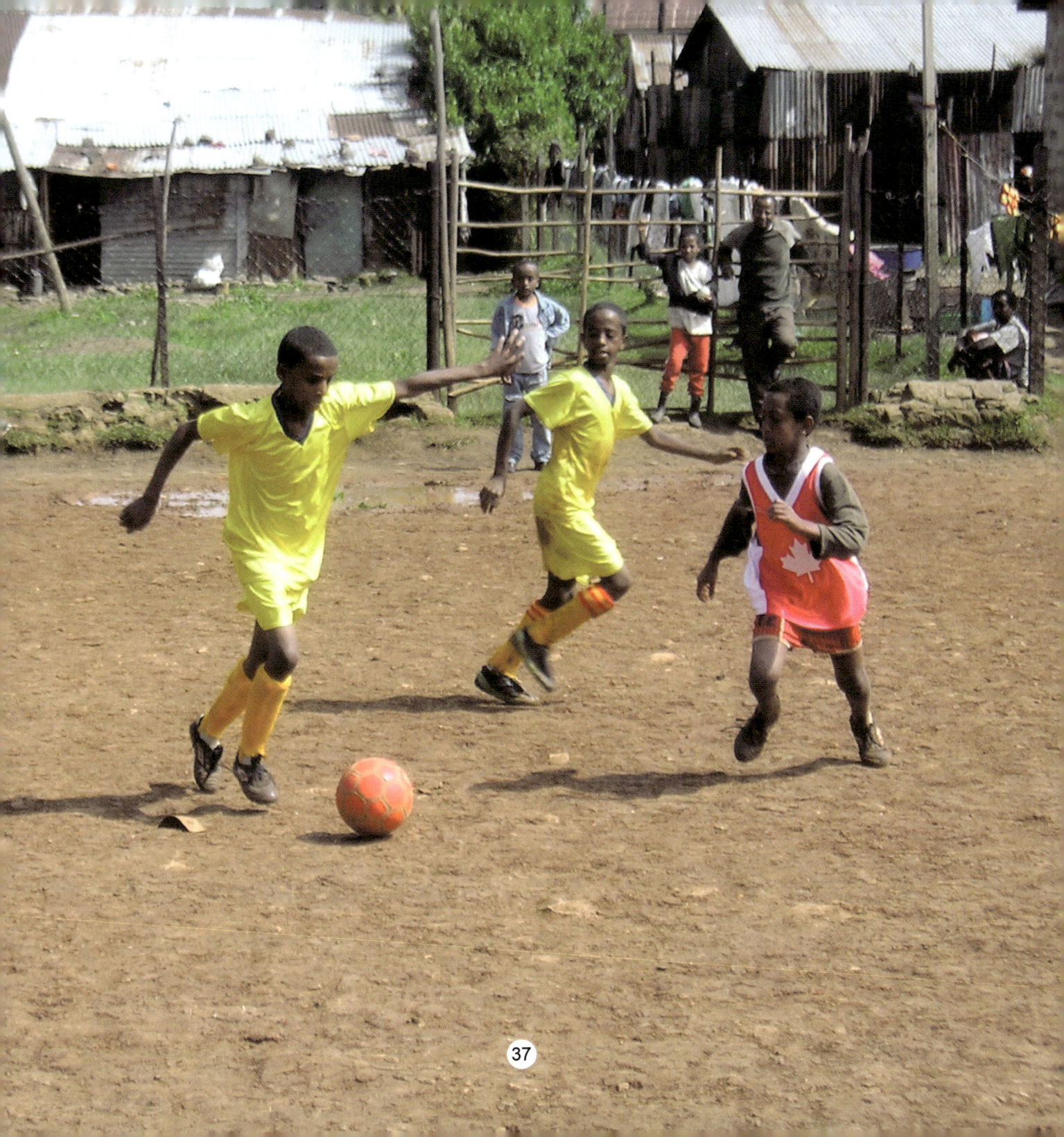

Inside Selamta Families

Chris:

After a couple of hours of soccer the sun started to set, and we headed back through the open fields, cleaning ourselves in muddy streams along the way. It struck me that most of these kids had years of experience using muddy streams to clean themselves. Robel and his brothers needed to return to their families for dinner. I went with Robel to his house for dinner, my first opportunity to see the houses of Selamta families.

Robel is clearly the man of his house. All of his siblings respect what Robel says, especially the younger boys. Robel ensured that his siblings were obedient and respectful of their mother. All of the children were intrigued by my iPod and couldn't stop listening to Usher, Chris Brown or Teddy Afro. Robel showed me around his house, an eight-room home with three bedrooms that was spotless. Two children slept together in each bed, and each child had their own drawer where their possessions were neatly placed and well taken care of.

In contrast to many American children, they didn't have much, but it was obvious that they valued and took care of their possessions. Their school clothes were neatly folded and cared for by the children. These children were grateful to have a roof over their heads, let alone a family place that they could call their home.

Robel told me about his Selamta family and a little about his life at Selamta.

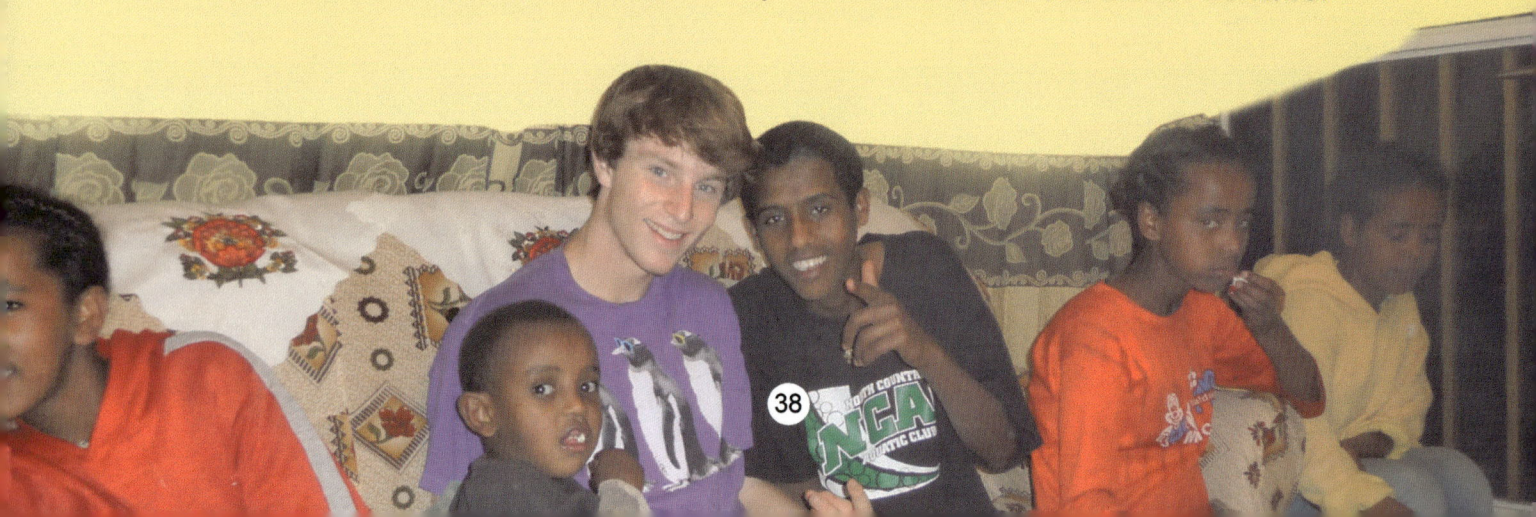

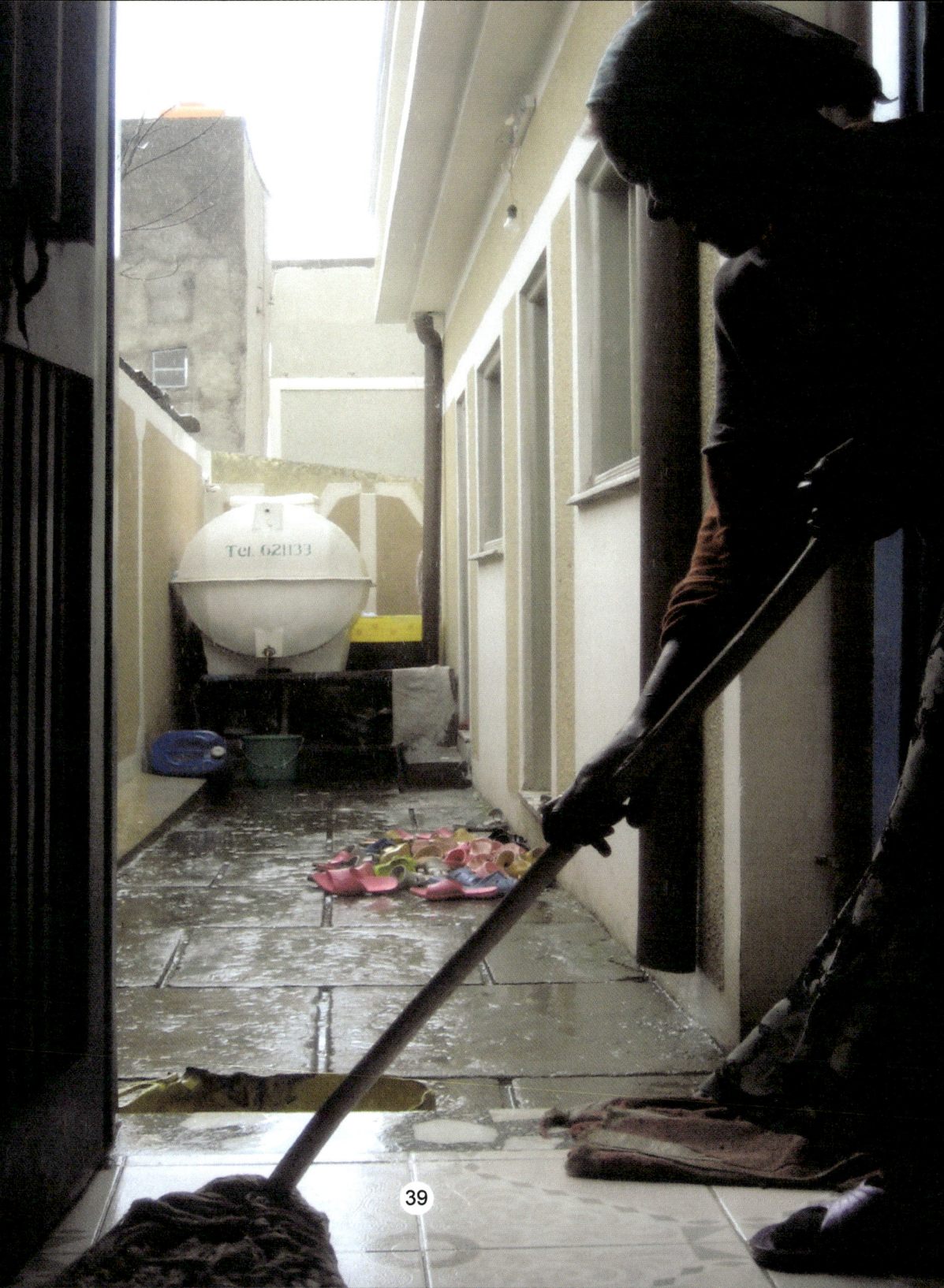

Robel:

In our house we have five boys and four girls. We have our mother, Selam, and an aunt called Roman. Out of the five boys, four of us sleep together in a room. Our room is just outside the main door within the compound. We get that room because I think that we are more grown up. The girls sleep inside the house. And our youngest brother, Yegermal, sleeps with our mother, Selam. My relationship with Yagarmall is special. We understand each other. He knows when I laugh or when I want to play. He also knows when I want to work, or when I want to just advise him. So we understand each other. When he asks me to read to him or tell him stories, I read to him. When I have some money to buy something, I sometimes buy some materials for him, and play with him.

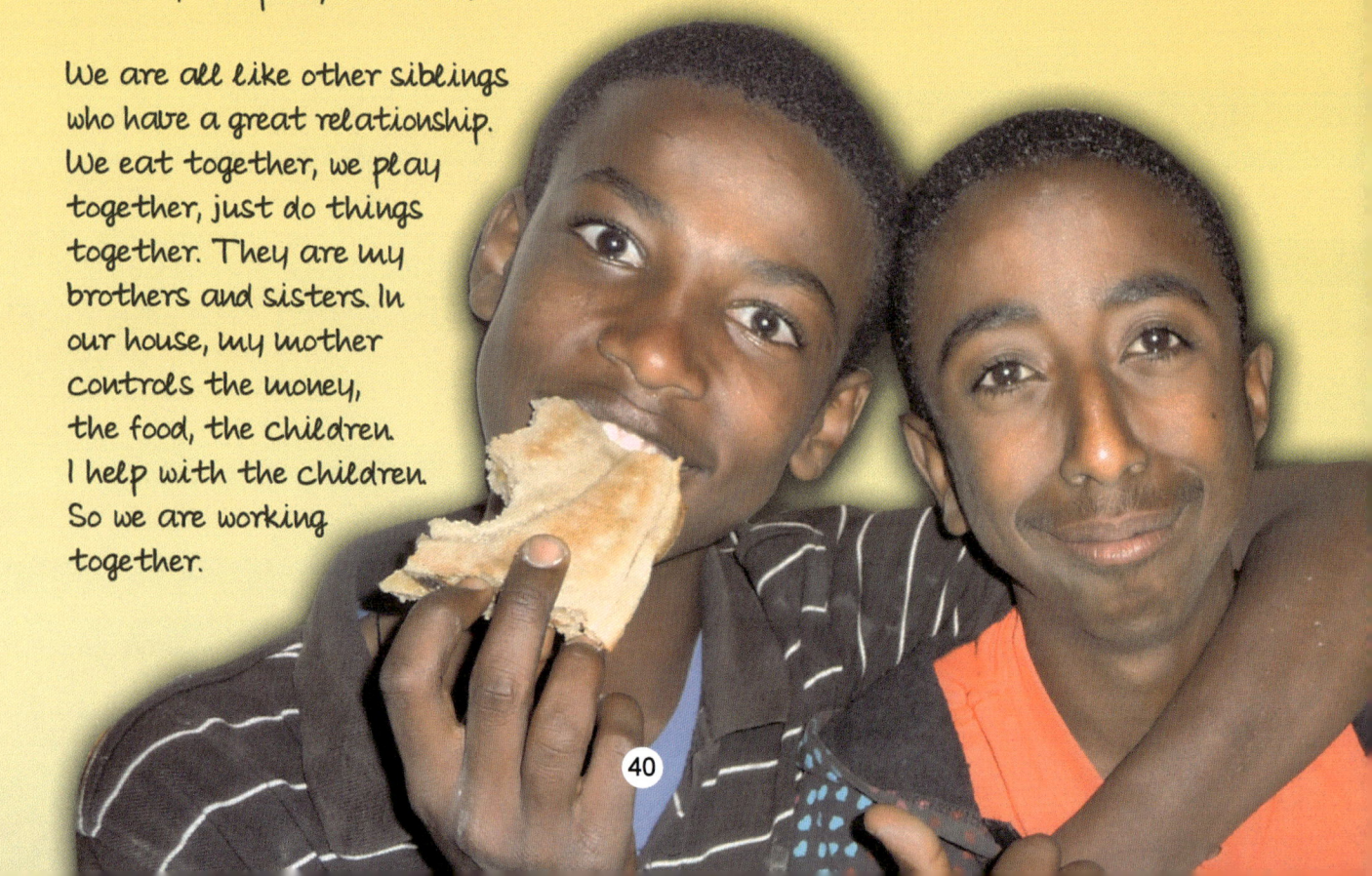

We are all like other siblings who have a great relationship. We eat together, we play together, just do things together. They are my brothers and sisters. In our house, my mother controls the money, the food, the children. I help with the children. So we are working together.

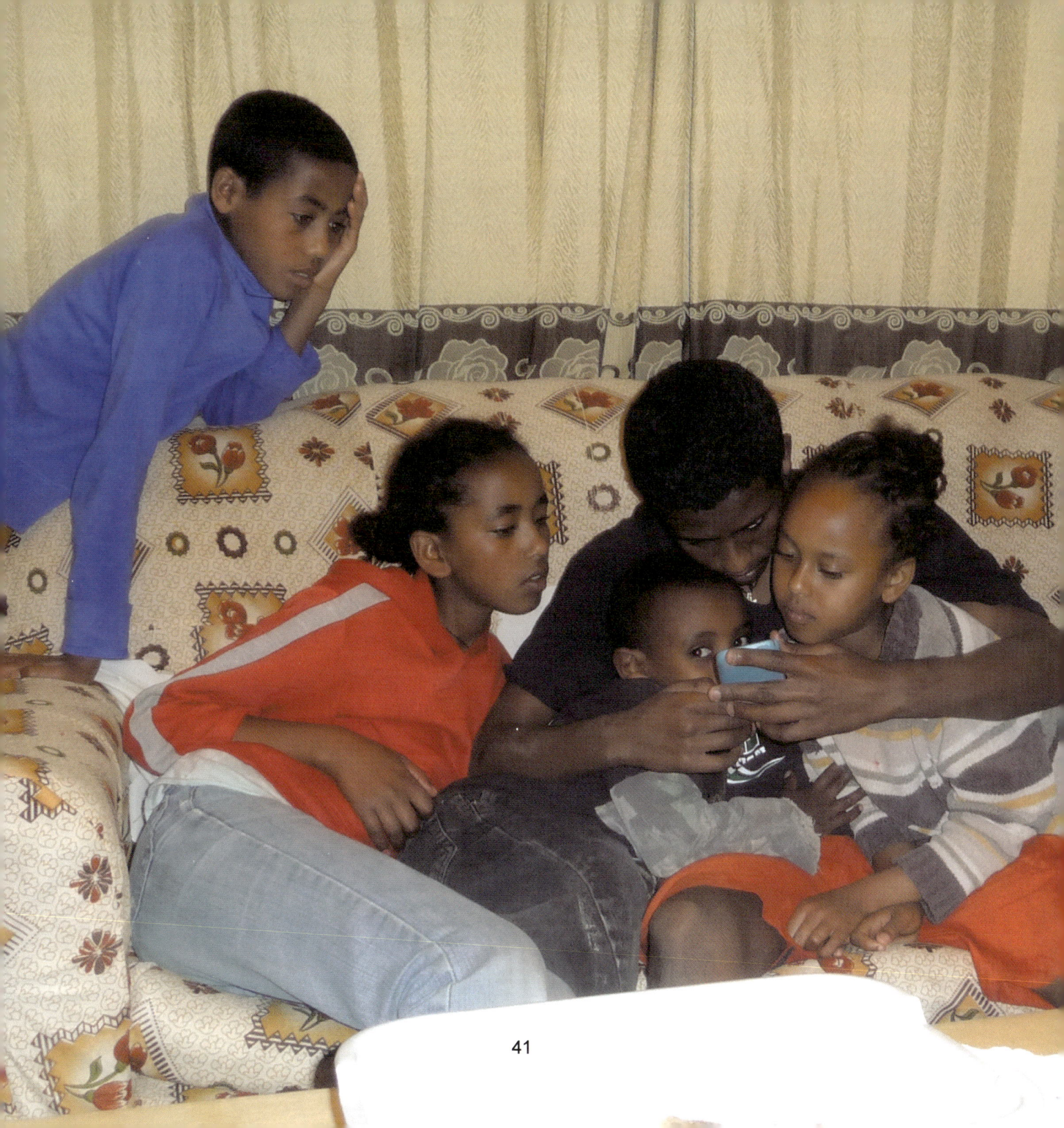

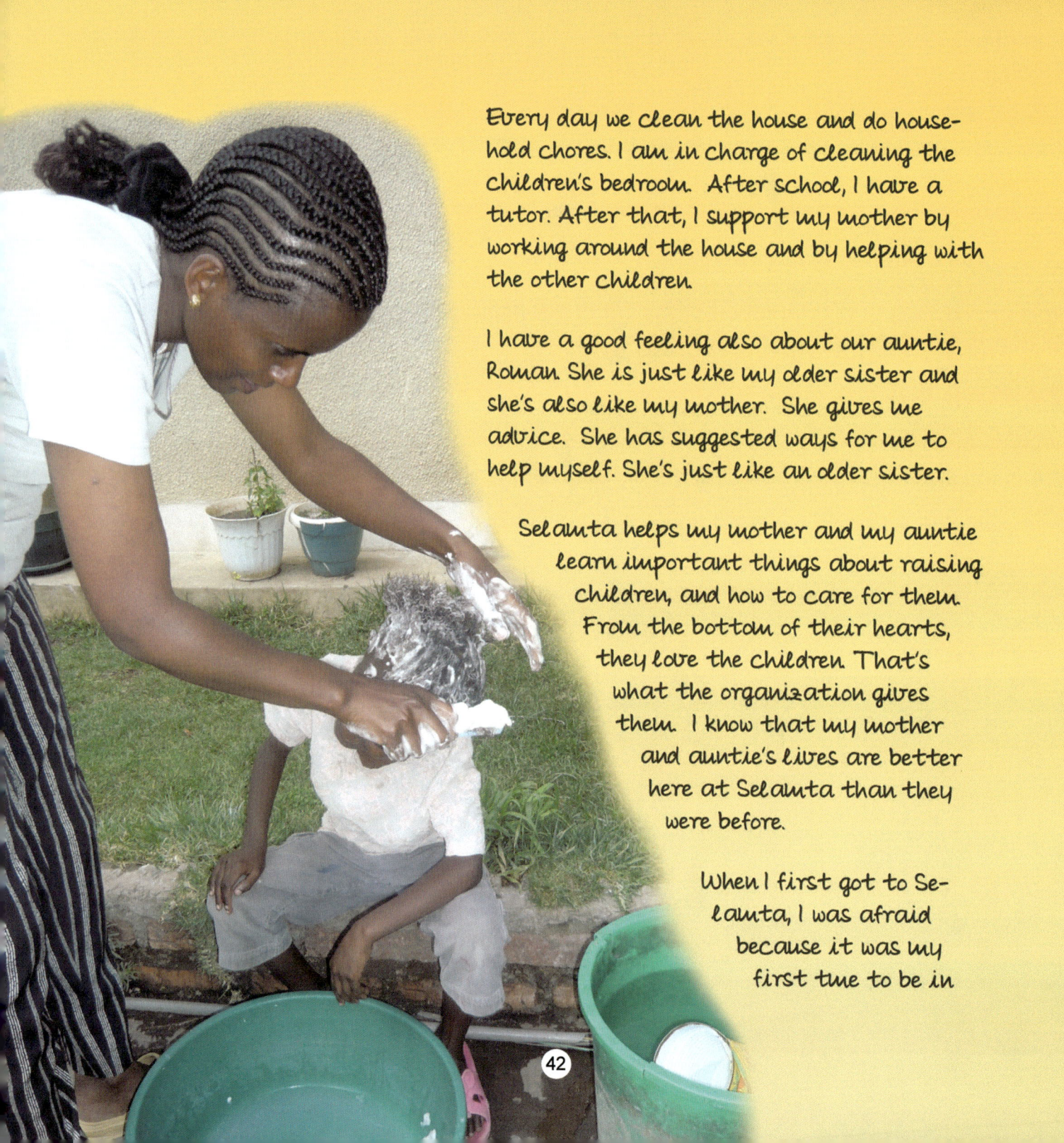

Every day we clean the house and do household chores. I am in charge of cleaning the children's bedroom. After school, I have a tutor. After that, I support my mother by working around the house and by helping with the other children.

I have a good feeling also about our auntie, Roman. She is just like my older sister and she's also like my mother. She gives me advice. She has suggested ways for me to help myself. She's just like an older sister.

Selamta helps my mother and my auntie learn important things about raising children, and how to care for them. From the bottom of their hearts, they love the children. That's what the organization gives them. I know that my mother and auntie's lives are better here at Selamta than they were before.

When I first got to Selamta, I was afraid because it was my first time to be in an organization. Then after a week, we joined the rest of the children. They gave me love. They included us and played with us, so I began to feel at home. The moms gave us special care. They always encouraged us to help ourselves. You have to help yourself to have a better life in the future.

There were some funny things that happened after we first arrived. At one of our first dinners they served us macaroni. It was white macaroni with white sauce. We had never had this before. We just sat and waited for them to serve the tomato sauce. They looked confused about why we weren't eating. Then they said, "Eat the macaroni."

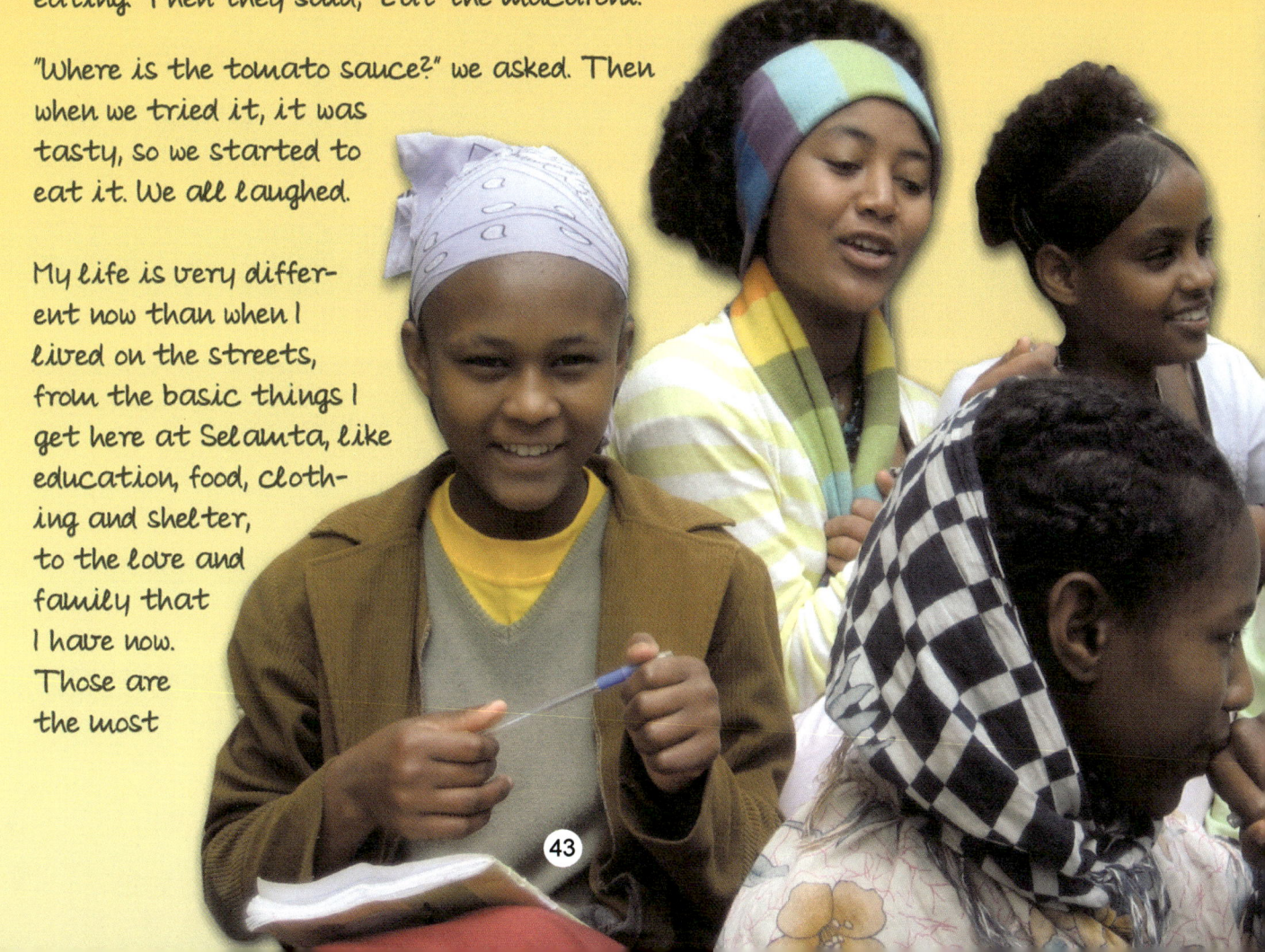

"Where is the tomato sauce?" we asked. Then when we tried it, it was tasty, so we started to eat it. We all laughed.

My life is very different now than when I lived on the streets, from the basic things I get here at Selamta, like education, food, clothing and shelter, to the love and family that I have now. Those are the most important things I found here at Selamta. I am always very happy to see new children come to Selamta because I know it's a new life for them. I sometimes pass on advice that was given to me. When they make mistakes, I guide them. I encourage them to do the right things here at Selamta because they have a chance at a new life. There are a lot of street children outside, so I want to help them just like we are helped here. It is impossible not to think about all of the children who still live on the streets.

Last year, I found my older brother, Tadessa. He was working as an assistant to the taxi drivers. He let me know that our younger brother was coming to Addis with our aunt because he had a water-borne disease. My older brother told me, "Masresha is here. He is sick. His whole body has some kind of allergy. He has got an itch in his body." He needed medication here in Addis. Tadesssa knew how much better Masresha's life would be at Selamta, and he asked me if I could help to get him here.

For a time, my aunt refused to give my brother to us. She needed Masresha to work for her. But Tadessa and I worked hard to convince her. We had all been separated for so long, and we wanted to be together again. "So why don't you give us our brother?" we asked. Then, at last, she gave us the child.

I was very, very happy to be reunited with my brother! It had been a very long time without him, and I never stopped thinking and worrying about him. Now he is part of our Selamta family, and I will never lose him again.

I talk about all of my ideas with my mother, Selam. Everything. When I see something wrong, or when I am in need of help, I just share my thoughts with her. She does a lot for me. She gives me advice to help myself. She's just like my real mom. I will never forget her.

45

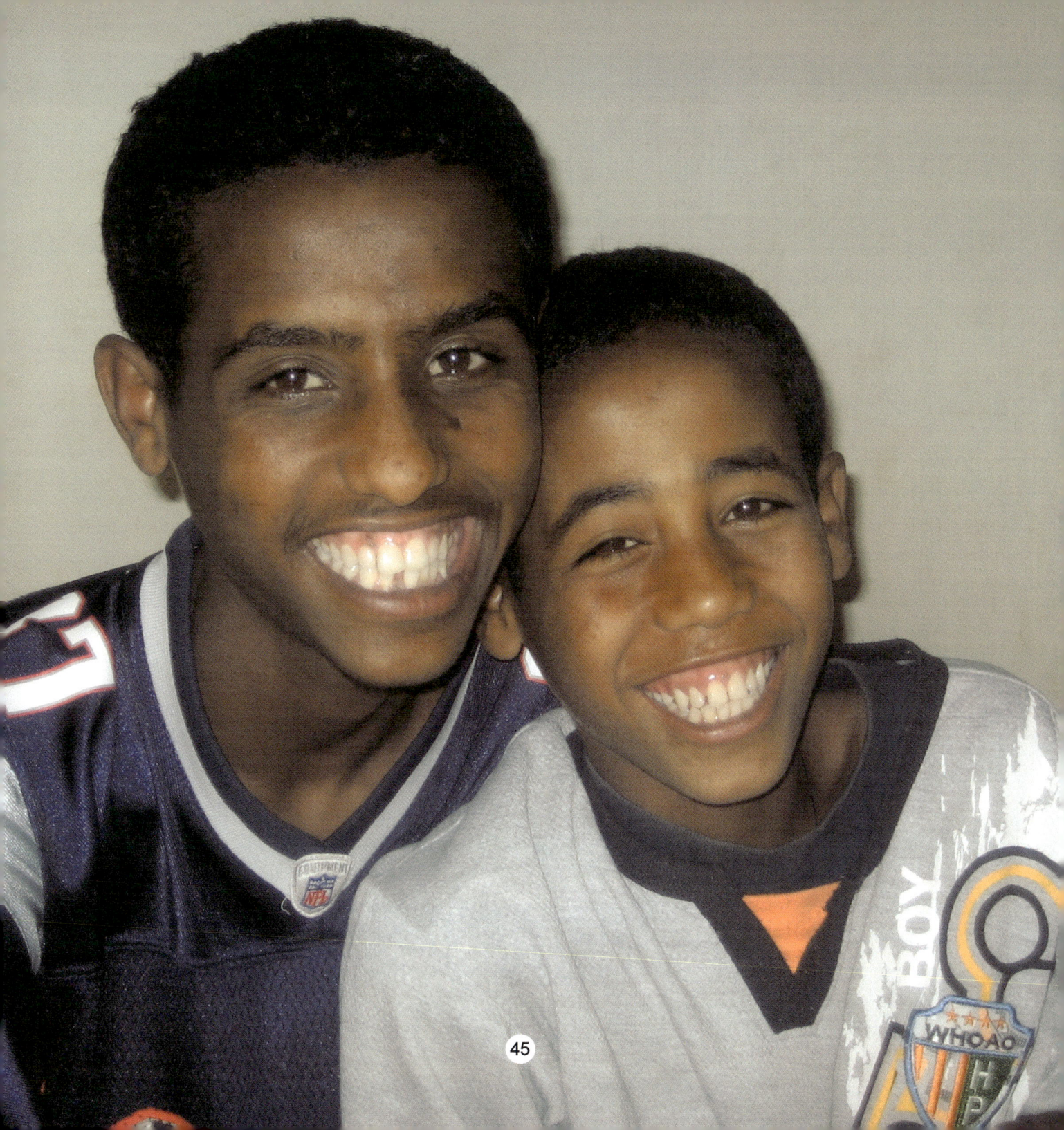

Some of my favorite times at Selamta are when we celebrate holidays together. The most special one was our Mother's Day celebration. All of us at Selamta have so much respect for the hard work of the mothers, so we were excited to celebrate Mother's Day. We had a cake and pizzas for everyone at the ceremony. The children all wrote poems for their mothers, and we read the poems during the party. It was our chance to give back to them.

When I am grown up, I will still always stay in touch with my mother, Selam and my other brothers and sisters. Even though my life may change, I will not take myself far away from them. I will always come here to be a part of their lives and help them as much as I can.

I will be happy if I can stay at Selamta for a long time. Our families are very loving. I don't know how far I will be able to go with my education, but I'll be happy to stay at Selamta until I finish my schooling.

If I had not been able to come to Selamta, I think I might be a father by now, and I would certainly not have an education. I might not have a good life. Family, for me, means a life full of love and peace, with respect for each other. That's family for me.

I give a special prayer for Selamta each night. It feels like home here. And the moms are very good. They're just like my mom, my real mom.

In the future, if I succeed I plan to adopt many children, especially the youngest ones. I am determined to help those children. The number of children I will adopt will depend on my finances, but the more money that I have, the more children I will adopt. I know others at Selamta feel the same way. We want to share with others the things that we have received.

Chris:

After dinner, and another coffee ceremony, I returned to the office with Robel and his brother. I gave them a flashlight and my iPod for the fifteen minute walk through the dark Ethiopian streets back to their home in Selamta. My thoughts drifted to the unlikely but miraculous reunion of Robel and his brother, and how full and rich their lives are in so many ways.

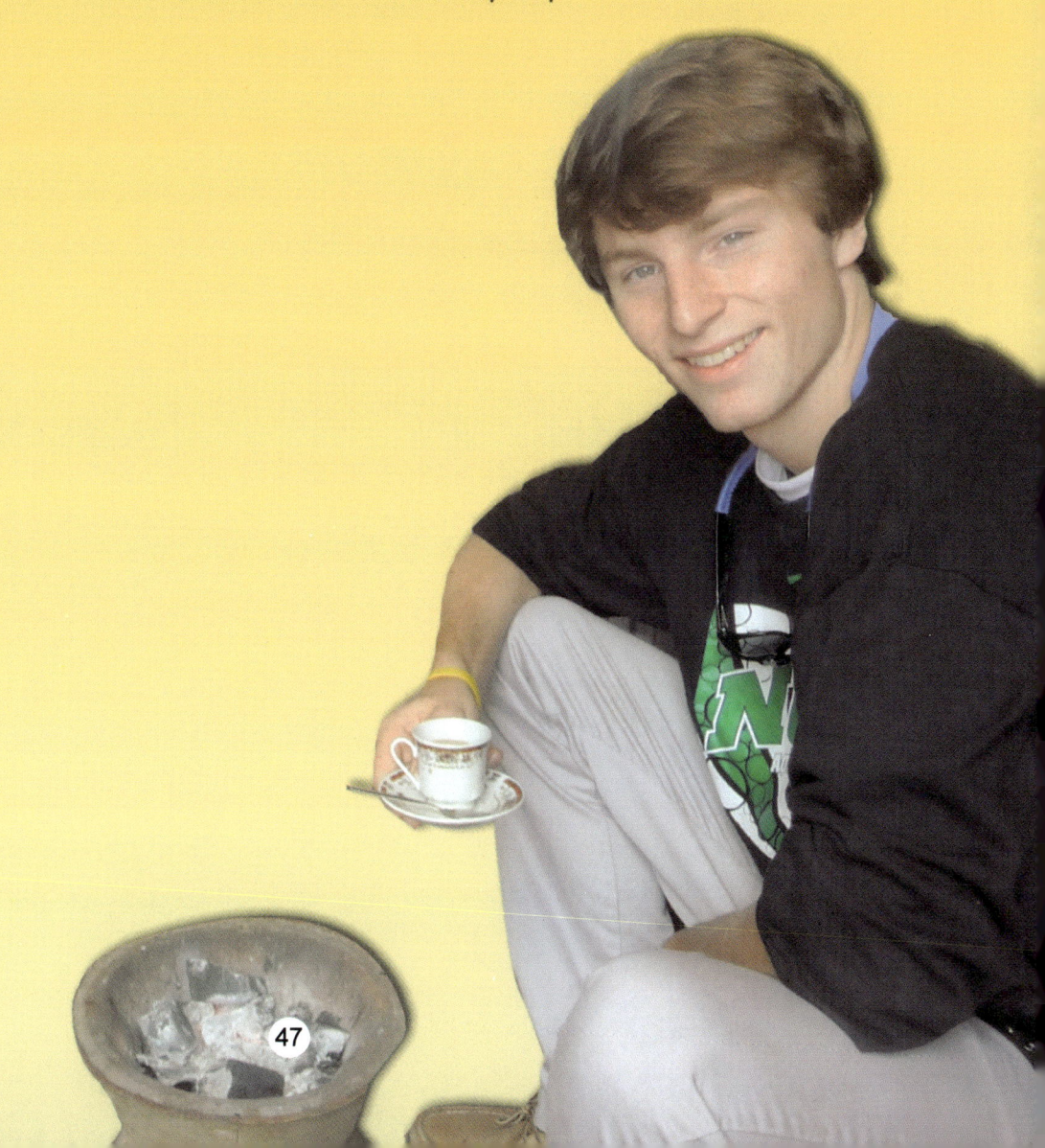

The Mercato

Chris:

Robel and I ventured out in the van to the Mercato. This is the largest open-air market in Africa, in the heart of Addis, a complex and immense area holding endless number of goods and countless people. Weaving through those streets in the new van, I feared that someone would hit us on these narrow passage ways they called streets.

We entered the Mercato on an uphill street on the car park section that was lined with random metal machines. We drove deep into the Mercato peering down alleyways filled with people and items. The horrible road conditions, ranging from back roads to highways, made it unclear what the van would run into. There could be a flock of sheep, a running bull, flooding or deep potholes anywhere along the streets. I hadn't really considered that the Selamta children had not grown up in cars as I had. Robel asked to stop the van, clearly having gotten sick from the experience of riding in a car.

The noise, the smell and the sun all contributed to the experience of being in the Mercato. We eventually found a place to park on the side of the road, next to a large lot of cars. In America I would have worried that a new car would get dinged, but here in Addis, this is not a priority. The number of people vastly outnumbered the number of cars—clearly most people came to the Mercato on foot. I felt like someone was always staring at me and watching my every move, and that I was inside another foreign place inside this already new world. Random people would approach me asking to have their picture taken with me with my camera.

There were shacks, stores, and vendors everywhere. Roads went from pavement to rocks to craters to mud pits. At any moment, I felt as if I were inches from being hit by a vehicle, animal or another person. Goats, dogs, cats, cows and donkeys roamed unleashed through the Mercato.

49

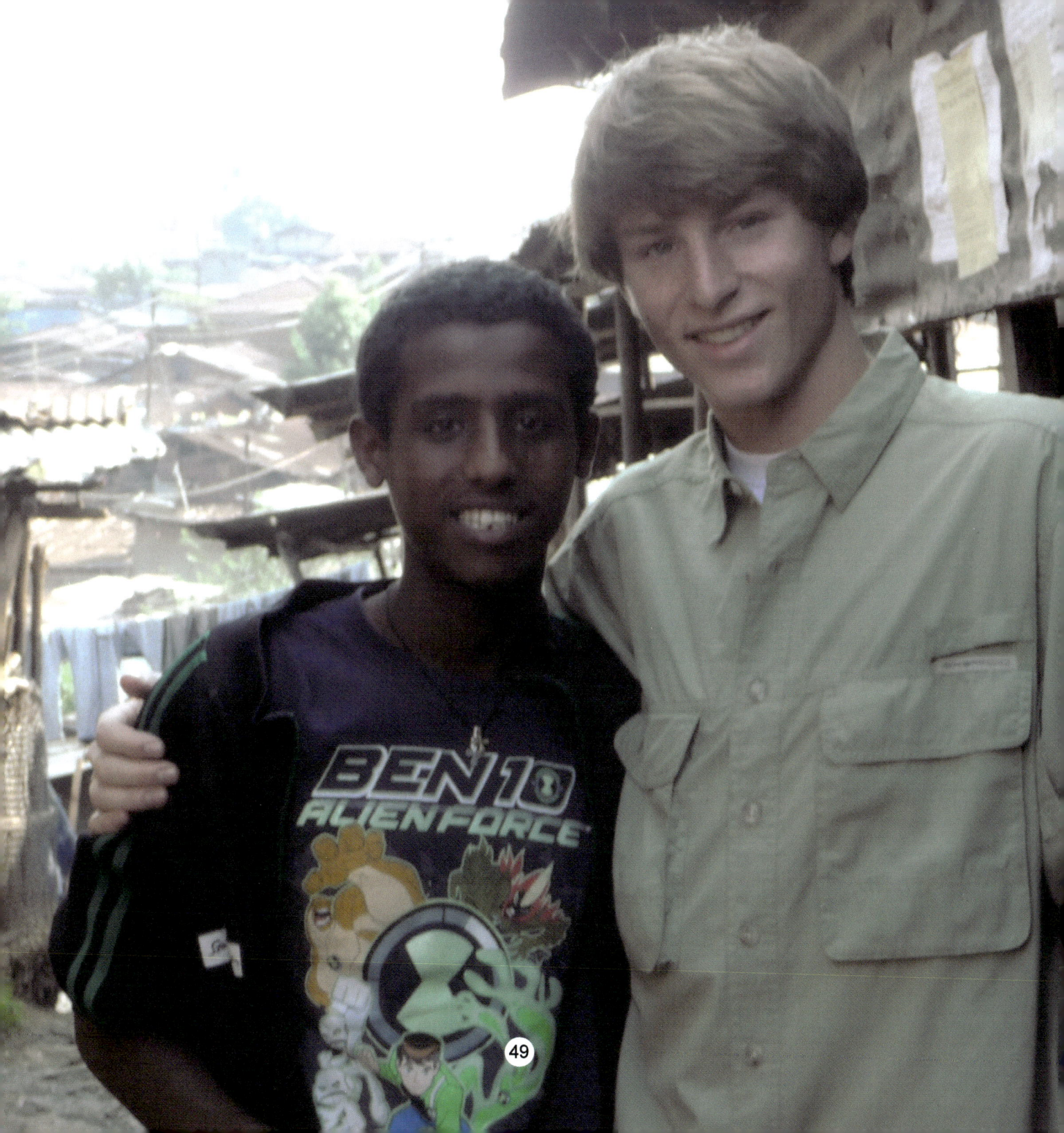

Many Muslims work at the Mercato, so at the holy hour most of the activity would abruptly stop. Most of the Mercato would shut down for several minutes and the religious prayer ceremonies would begin.

Moving from section to section of the Mercato, I noticed that the merchandise would change from shoes to spices to metal, and everything in between.

Robel:

We saw a lot of things in the Merkato. Different, amazing things, like people who cut cans or irons into other things. Stuff they are doing at the Merkato was very amazing for us. Not only for Chris but for me, too.

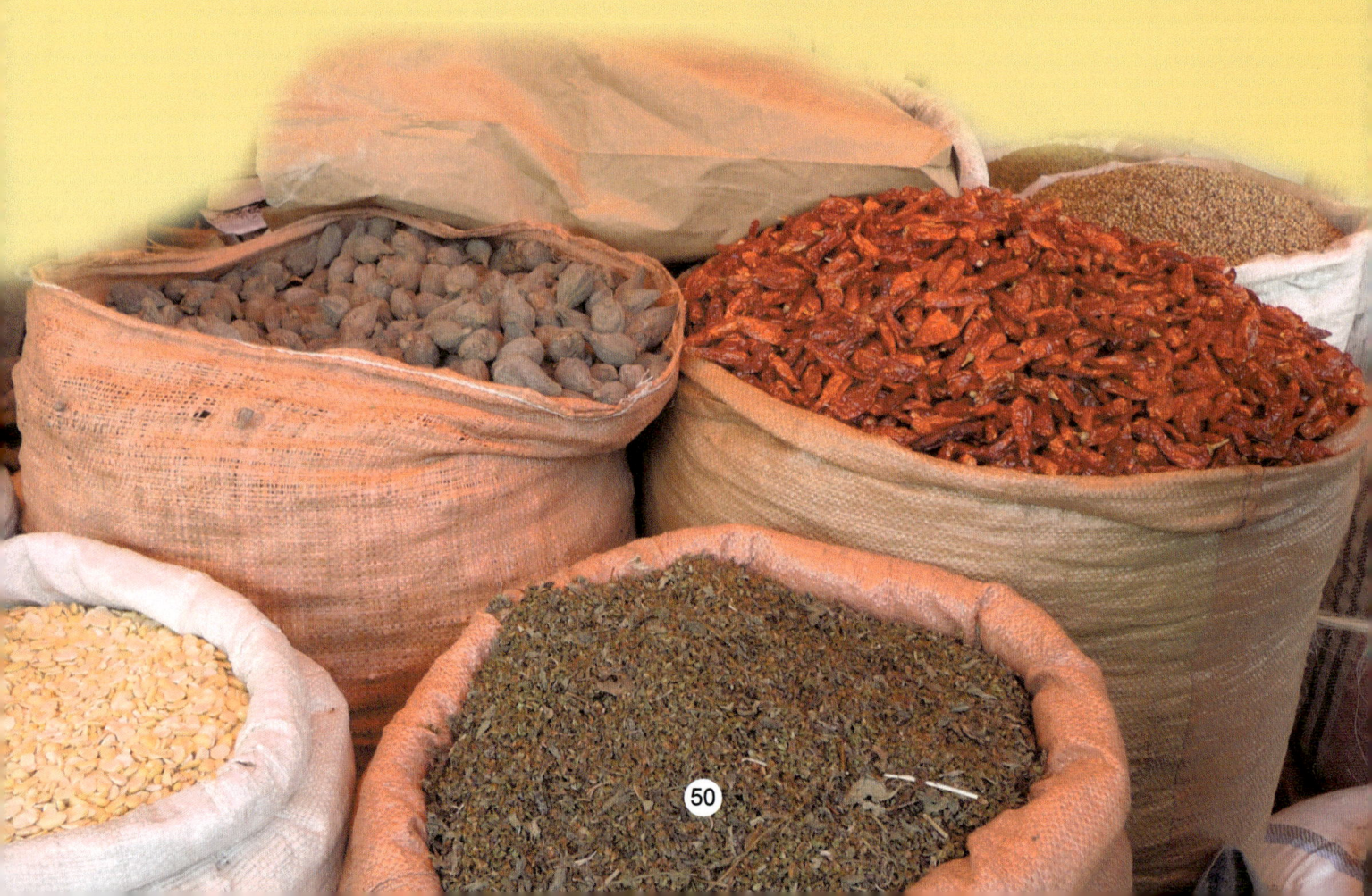

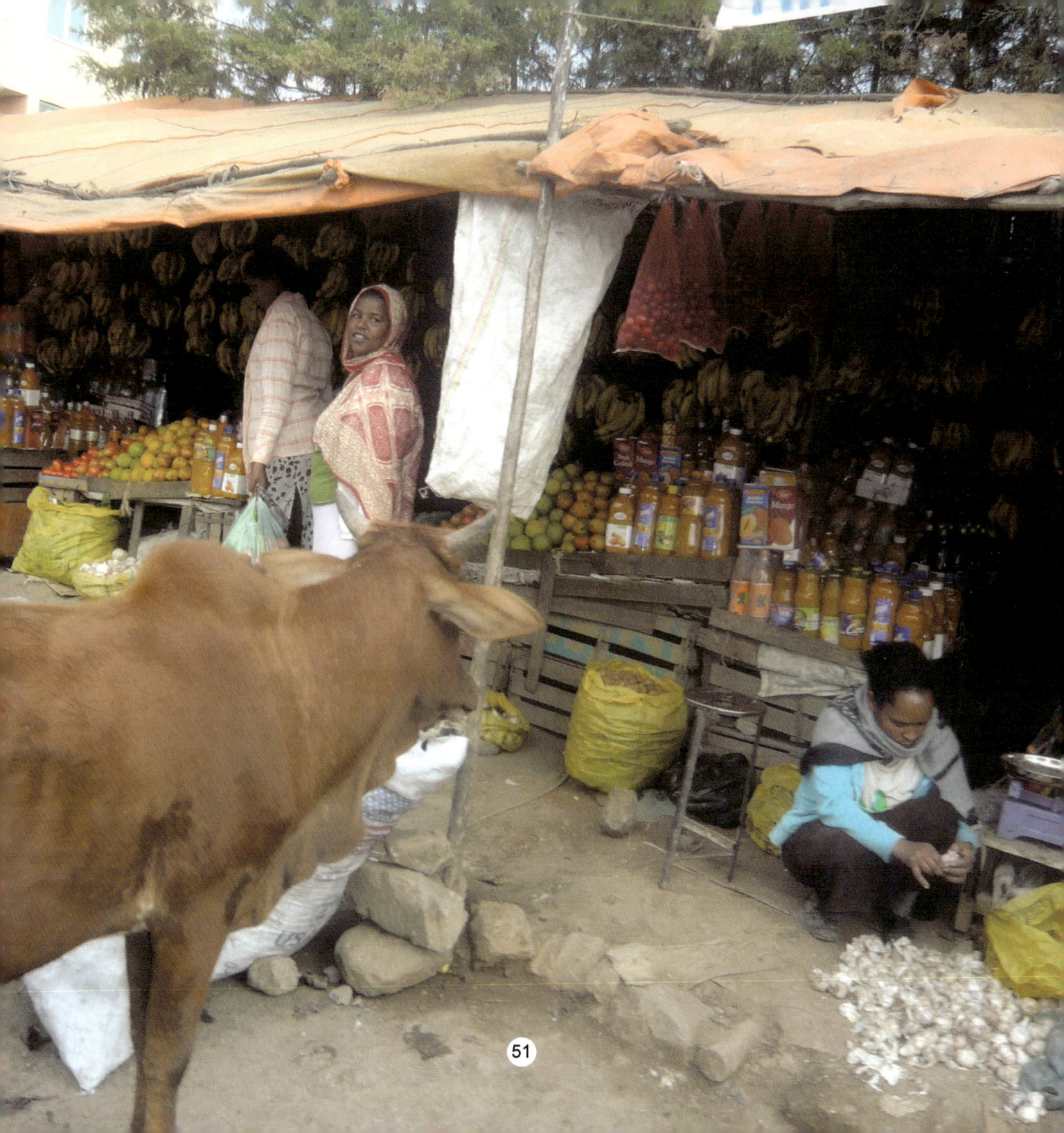

School

Chris:

As we drove, we talked. Robel told me about his school and his education. I listened and recognized how different it had been in so many ways from my own.

Robel:

When I first started school at The Alpha School, many of the subjects were taught in English. That was new for me. Especially general sciences and social studies, they were all in English. School was, at first, very difficult for me. I was very discouraged. But after a month or so, I started to work harder and got better results. I went to the Alpha School. It is a private school but private schools are very different than in the United States. The tuition is $10 a month. I thought it was a good school. I hope if I do well that I will have a chance to get a scholarship or to continue my education by going to college.

I didn't have a chance to go to school before the Alpha School, but when I lived on the streets we sometimes went to a place called Hope Enterprise. They would give us tea with bread, and then they gave us some courses in English. They taught us the letters and things like that. I started writing and learning spelling then. My favorite courses now are music and physics. I have a talent for music. At school we learn about music and the history of music in Ethiopia.

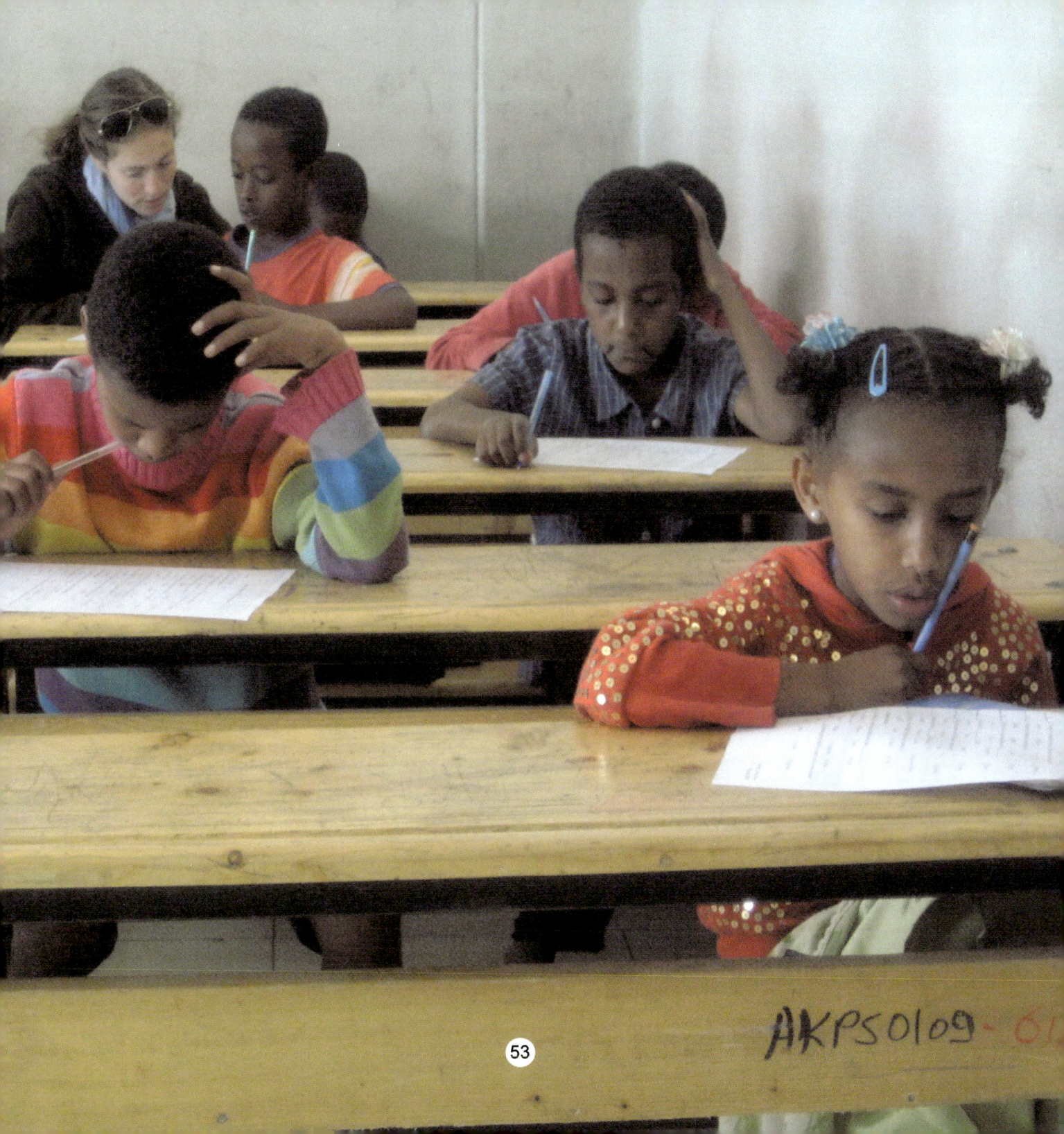

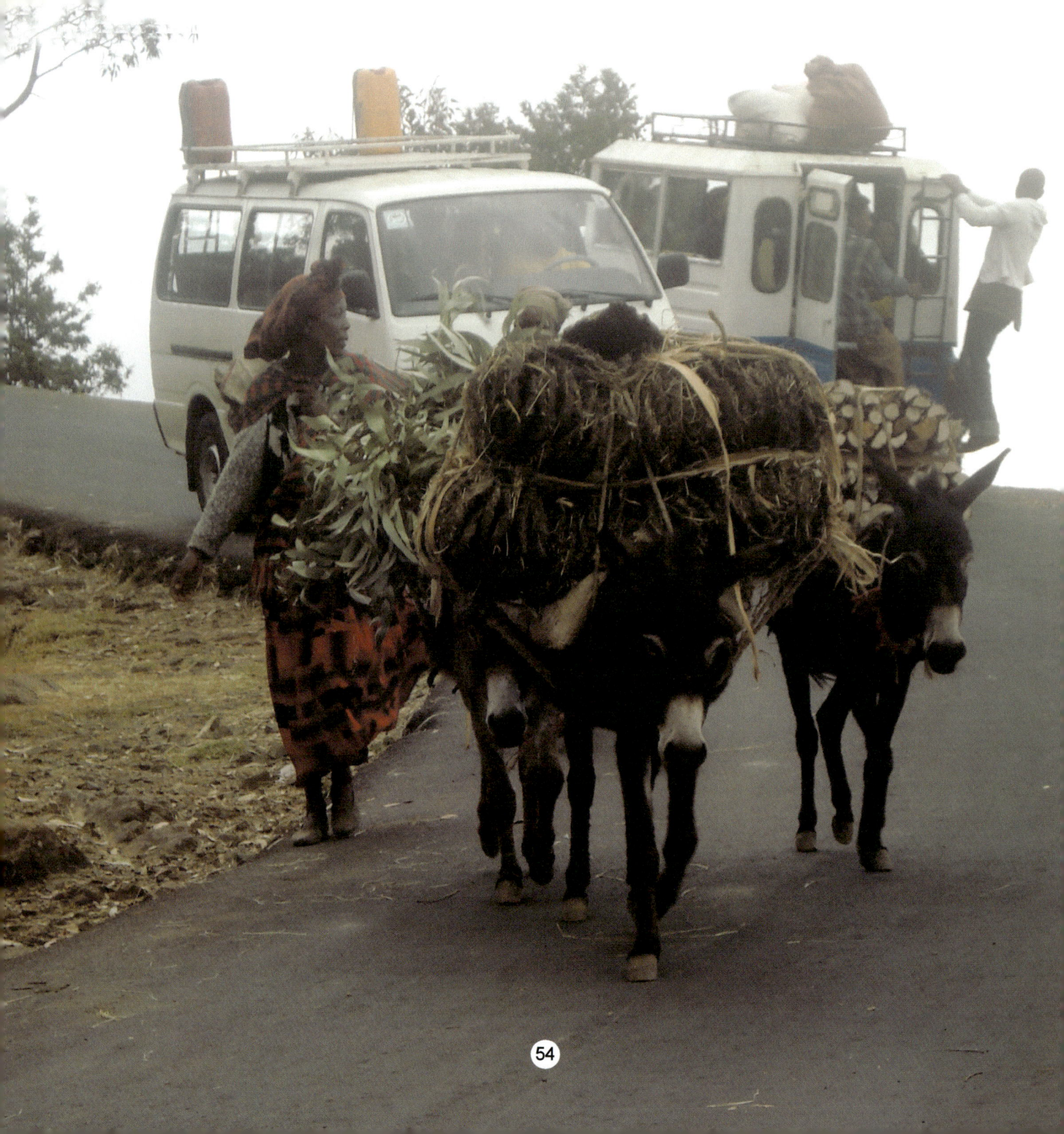

Entoto

Robel:

I was glad that we had the chance to see Entoto Mountain. It is an important part of Ethiopia's history. I had heard about Entoto before, but I hadn't had the experience to go there. My first chance to visit this piece of our history was with Chris. I was glad that I had learned a lot about the place, the palaces, and the stories that start at Entoto.

Chris:

Considering my relatively brief stay in Addis I wanted to make the most of each and every day. I had heard about a church and palace on top of the surrounding mountains, but I did not know where it was, or how to get there. We hopped in the van and headed to Entoto.

Entoto was the palace of the late King Menelik, and dates back from the time of the colonization of Africa. Ethiopians are very proud that Ethiopia is one of a few countries to never be ruled by a European power. The Italians during the late 1800's tried to overpower and colonize Ethiopia like so many other European powers had previously tried to do. King Menelik, and Queen Taitu thankfully kept the Italians out of Ethiopia, but it was the next emperor, Haile Selassie, who finally ensured Ethiopia's independence. It was fascinating to see this early African Emperor's palace atop one of tallest mountains surrounding Addis. There was a small museum at the top of the mountain where we were given a brief history lesson about the area, but we were not allowed to take pictures. After a few hours of checking all the thatch-roofed buildings and mud made walls, we headed back to Addis.

56

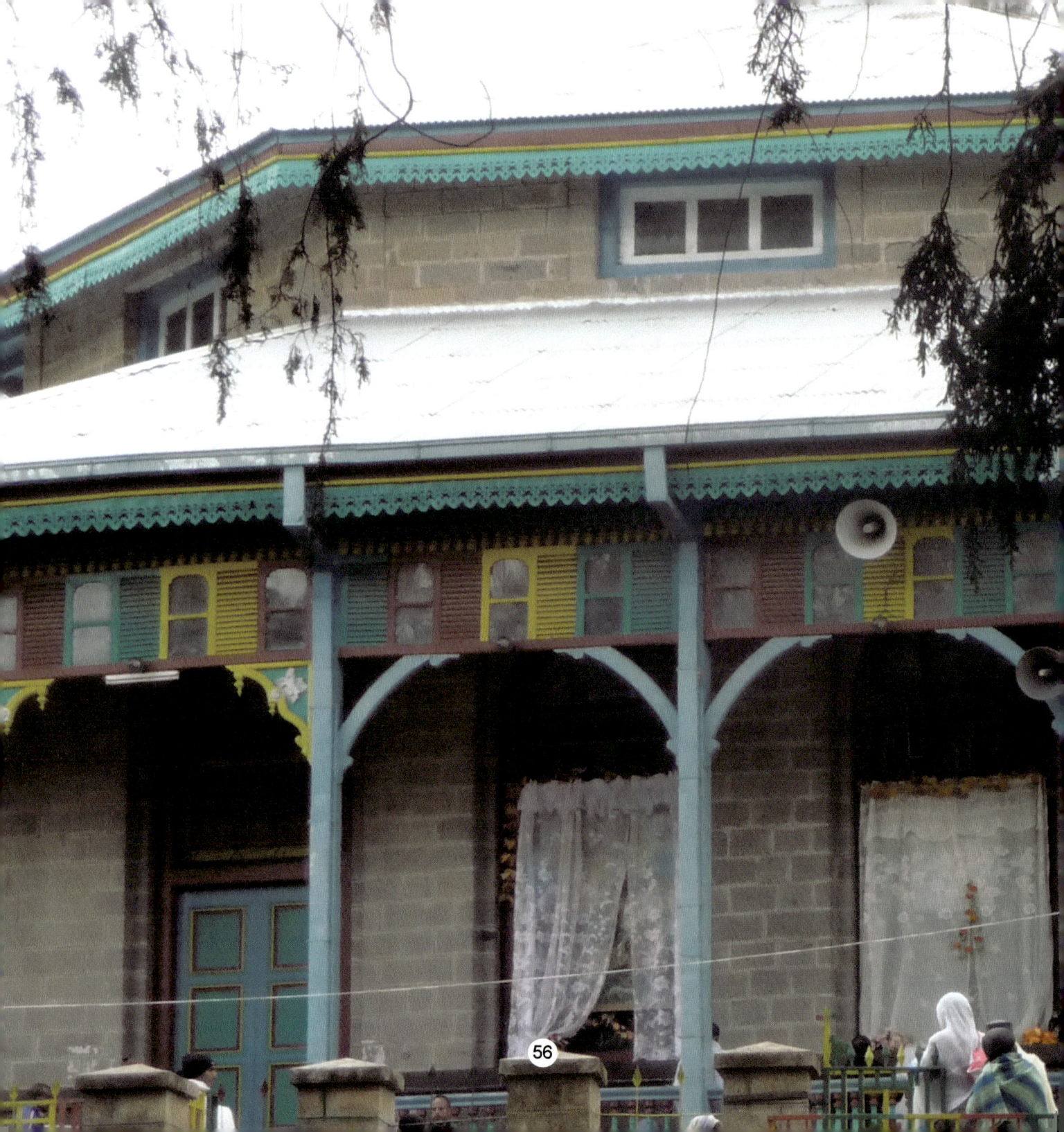

57

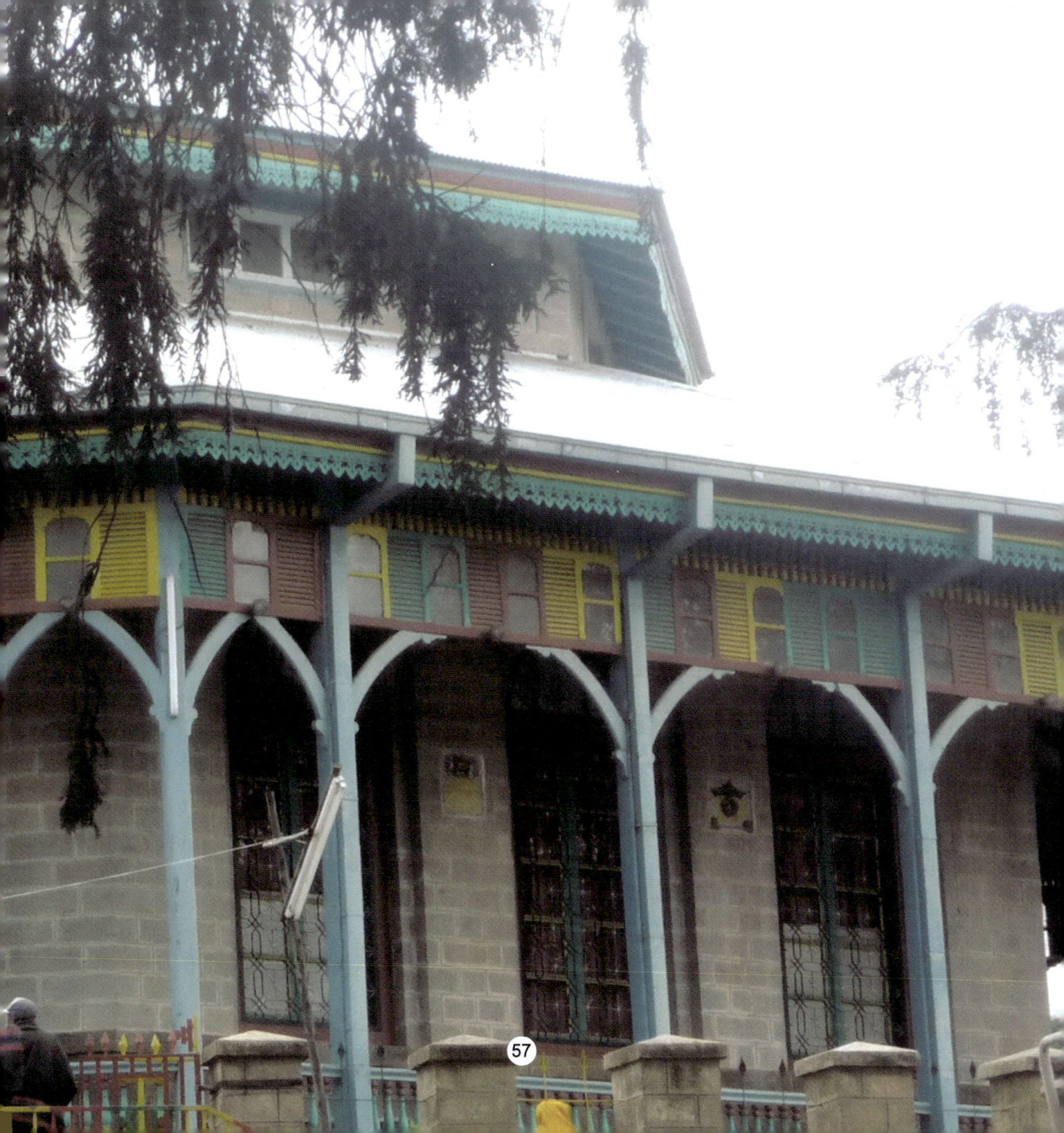

Chris:

On our descent to Addis there were a few clearings where you could see all of Addis. Being the tourist that I was, I had to get this picture. While standing to the side of the road there were occasional cars that would pass and a few children running around on the steep mountainside. I decided to take a picture of two children who were talking in a shallow cave. These children immediately popped up and ran towards me to see what I was up to. Shortly afterwards another boy or two came, this time carrying a whip, the large type of cracking whip that is used to move animals, to try and teach me how to use it. All of this happened very quickly.

Initially there were just five or six kids who were asking for money and saying hello, but this all changed very quickly. As soon as I took some money out of my pocket I heard Robel tell me to put it away, and he quickly pointed to a mob of children running towards me.

What started as another friendly encounter with some street children, turned into a small brawl on the side of a mountain, with kids tearing at me and screaming for money. I have no idea where all these kids came from, but it seemed as though they literally popped out of the ground or fell from the sky. I recognized that this was not a safe situation, and things were getting out of control quickly. I grabbed Robel by the arm and we had to fight our way out of the crowd and sprint to the van in a hurry. After jumping in the van, kids grabbed the window and banged on the side, some even hung on and cried, begging for some money. This was one of the only two times I felt unsafe in Ethiopia. It was my fault for bringing out money when I didn't fully understand my surroundings.

My trip to Entoto was a great way to learn some history of Ethiopia and get a chance to see a little more than just urban Addis. I thought that I would be most taken with the brief history lesson about Ethiopia, but what I remember

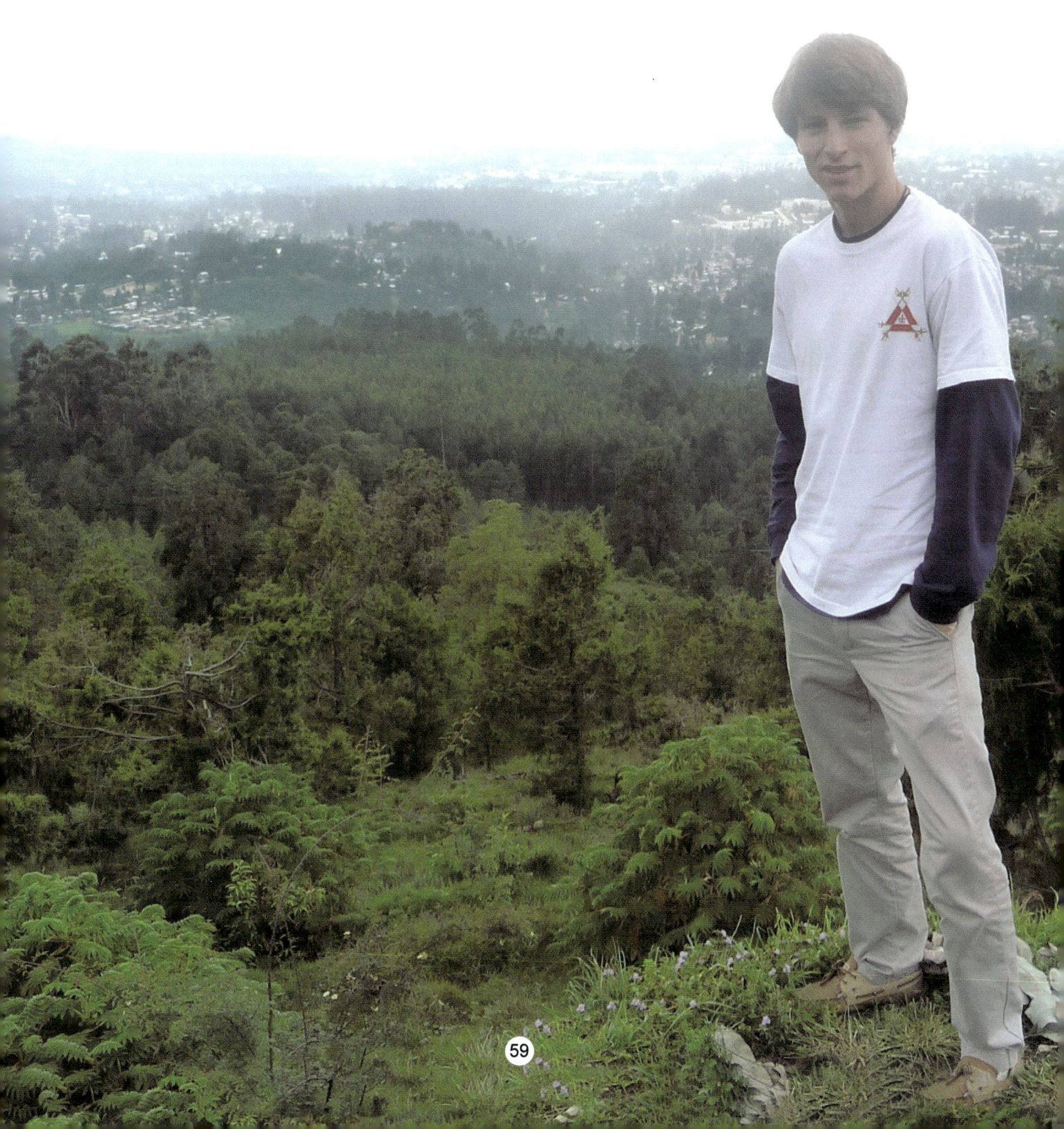

most was being confronted at the lookout. Witnessing these desperate, rag covered children was yet another humbling experience. As I ran toward the van that day, I dropped on the ground all of the money in my pockets--around 200 birr. I wonder what that money was used for by those children--was it for food, clothes, maybe even a toy? Or is it buried within the cave where those children lived, being saved for a time that becomes even more desperate? Or was it all torn apart between the mob of children that day? I will never know the answer to these questions, but I continue to wonder, and hope that it brought some of those children, a small sliver of happiness.

Robel:

When we were at Entoto some beggars surrounded Chris and demanded money. He had followed one child and gave him 50 birr. Then all of a sudden a lot of children were all around him, and he had a very confused look on his face. That was a shocking moment for me. I asked them to let him free. They even started to ask me for money, too. I tried to separate him from the children. Then we quickly got into the van. It was a little bit frightening.

I realized how far I had come from the days that I might have been part of a group like that. I felt frightened and confused. There was so much that Chris did not understand in that situation, I felt protective of him.

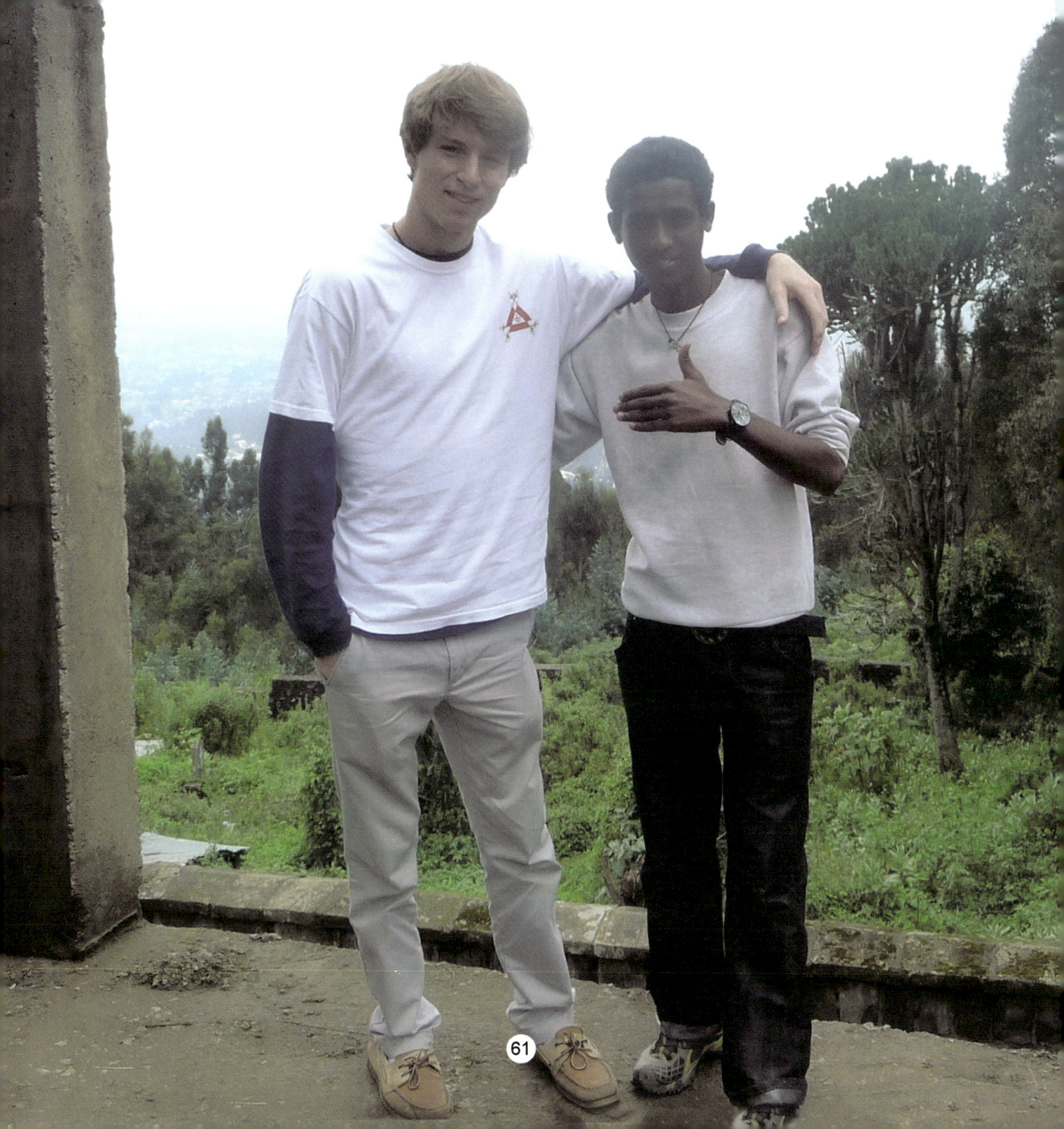

Life on the Streets

Chris:

Robel and I visited many places together and laughed a lot as we explored the area, but the trip we took so that Robel could share his life on the streets with me was very different. It was clear that he was sharing with me memories that he often keeps hidden away to protect himself from the pain that they bring. I was honored that he cared enough about me to trust me to share this part of his past. He had lived on the streets for five years, but Kasanches is the place where he lived for four of those years.

I worried that coming back would be difficult for Robel. I saw on his face how much of an impact it had on him to return to his old life. I could only imagine all the feelings he must have had. He lived on the streets of Kasanches with different kids at different times during those years. As we walked around, Robel pointed out his "home." We walked down a dirt path with a stream coming down the hill over the rocks, garbage and mud. We suddenly stopped at about a one foot wide piece of concrete that jutted out from a wall and ran the entire length of the wall on the side of the road.

Robel explained that there had been a low wall on one side that had been knocked down since he had left for Selamta. He would run a tarp from the high wall to the low wall, and he and the other kids would lie single file under the tarp on the concrete. To me, it looked like a wrecking ball had just passed, but I realized that this "home" helped to shape Robel into such a compassionate man who wanted so much to rescue other street children and offer his guidance.

We then walked up the street several blocks until we reached a path leading down to a bridge to cross into back alleys through Addis. There was a river under the bridge, and Robel pointed out where he would bathe. We went down to the river, and I recognized that the brown piles of "mud" were actually human waste. Clearly, this river is still used as a bathing spot during the non-rainy season. The rain makes the water more polluted, and the street children know not to bathe in it during those times in order to avoid water borne diseases. I was shocked to see the muddy river that was used almost daily by thousands of Ethiopian children. I was happy that Robel now lived at Selamta in a house with plumbing.

We then walked down an alley where he would gather his food. Bags of food would be tossed out into the streets, and kids would swarm around the bags in search of their next meal. I stopped when I saw four or five boys encircling one of these bags, eating whatever was inside. Just three years ago, Robel had been one of those boys.

As we kept walking, Robel ran into some of his old street friends. They quickly chatted, but as fast as they appeared, they were suddenly gone. Robel told me that one of these kids had actually tried to join an orphanage, but lasted in it for only one week. Orphanages do not allow children who are addicted to cigarettes, alcohol or chewing "chat." Chat is a form of a cocoa leaf. Kids use alcohol and cigarettes in order to keep themselves warm, and to stay awake in order to fight off any predators. It struck me how unfair this system is to these kids who are already at such a disadvantage.

Robel:

When I went back to the place where I lived for so long on the streets, I felt overwhelmed. I tried not to cry, but I couldn't keep the tears back. This was the place I used to live and sleep before. This was the place by the waters where I tried to find food, tried to stay safe, tried to survive. I remember the hunger, the fear, and the desperation. Thinking of my past life made me so sad.

From the look on Chris' face, I knew that he understood and felt as sad about my past life as I did. I could see it in his expression. For me, a true friend is just like a brother who shares the most important things with you. And you share a lot of things with him. Chris is more than a friend to me. I call him my brother. Even though we have different skins, we are brothers.

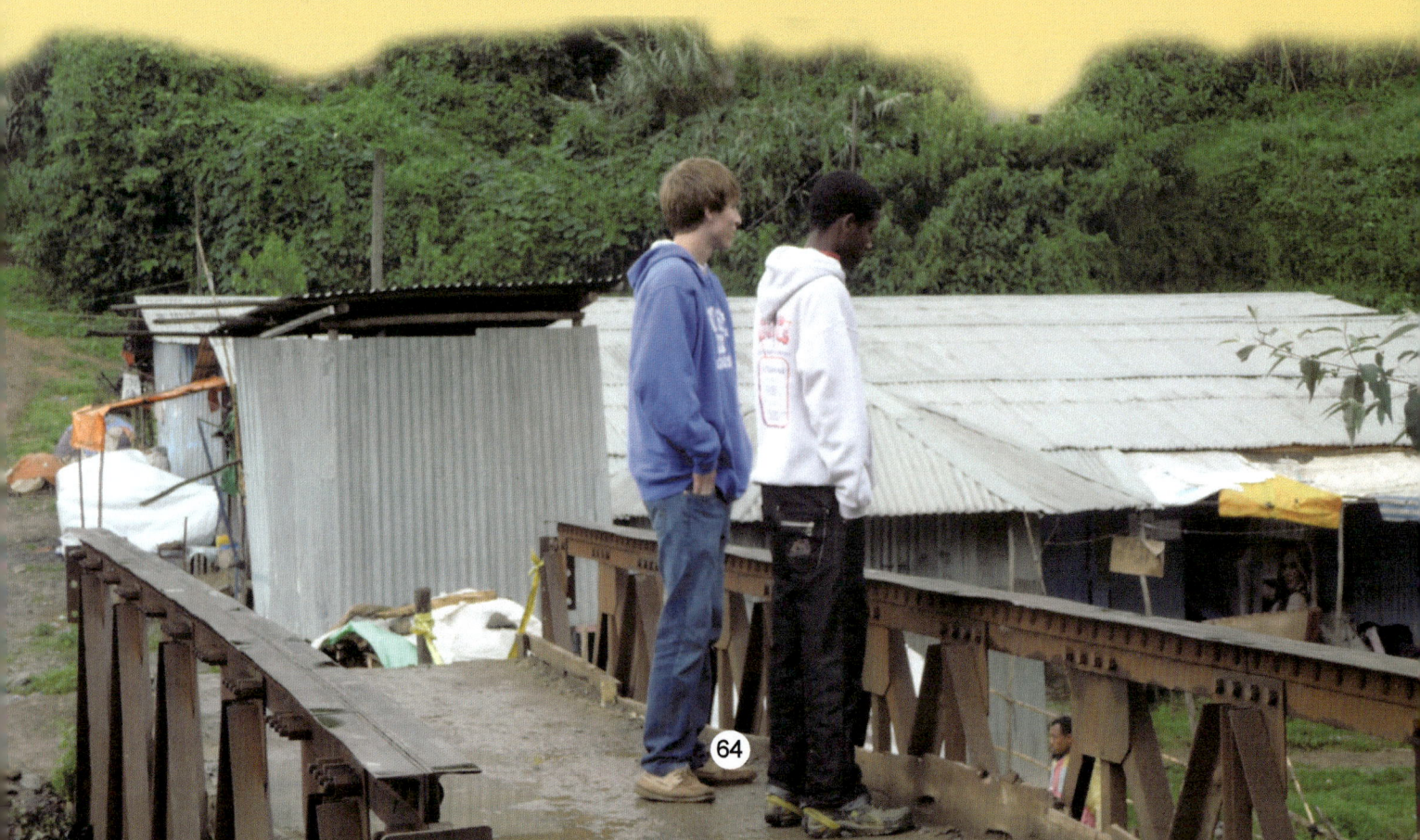

When I lived on the streets, some of the other kids were older than me, and some were younger. They taught me how to survive. It is hard to describe how dangerous some of the things that happen on the streets are. When you live on the streets, drunk men or robbers might force you to do horrible things. They would rape us or hurt us and things like that. We tried to control as much of our world as we could as kids. We watched out for each other.

Most of the time kids fell into bad habits and started to do things like smoking, stealing, and gambling. After I got away from the street life, I regretted what I did before. We learned bad things.

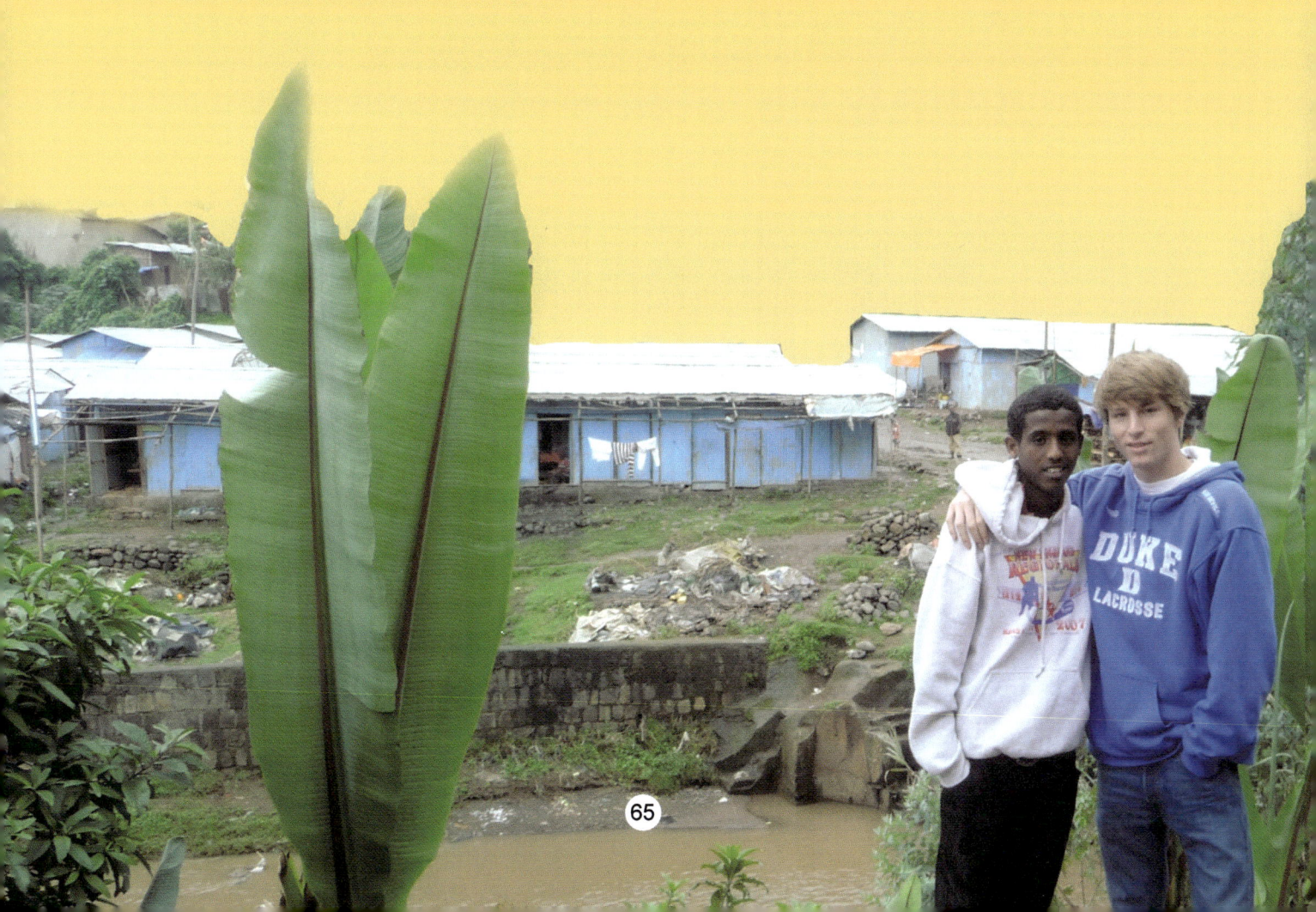

There were reasons for some of the bad habits we developed. Some kids smoked because it was so cold at night. They felt that smoking protected them from the cold. They also believed that smoking keeps you stimulated so you will not sleep the whole night. We learned to sleep during the daytime when we could because during the nighttime there were a lot of problems like drunk men or gangs or robbers. It's much more dangerous during the night, so we would try to stay awake and walk around the city. Then we would get tired and sleep. That's why the kids smoked cigarettes. And also to feel good, warm.

It was always the same, what we did for the whole week. When we woke up from sleep in the morning, the first thing we did was search for food. Breakfast. Then after we found food, we just started trying to carry things for people for money. It might be different things. It might be only a sack, or it might be tef, it might be maize. We carried different things from the taxis or the busses. We carried things to people's houses. Then after we got money, we would go to watch movies. We would go to these small movie houses that used a kind of television to show movies. Then after the sunset, we'd get out from the movie house and we would try to find some scraps of chat to chew from the trash, leftover chat. We chewed it.

67

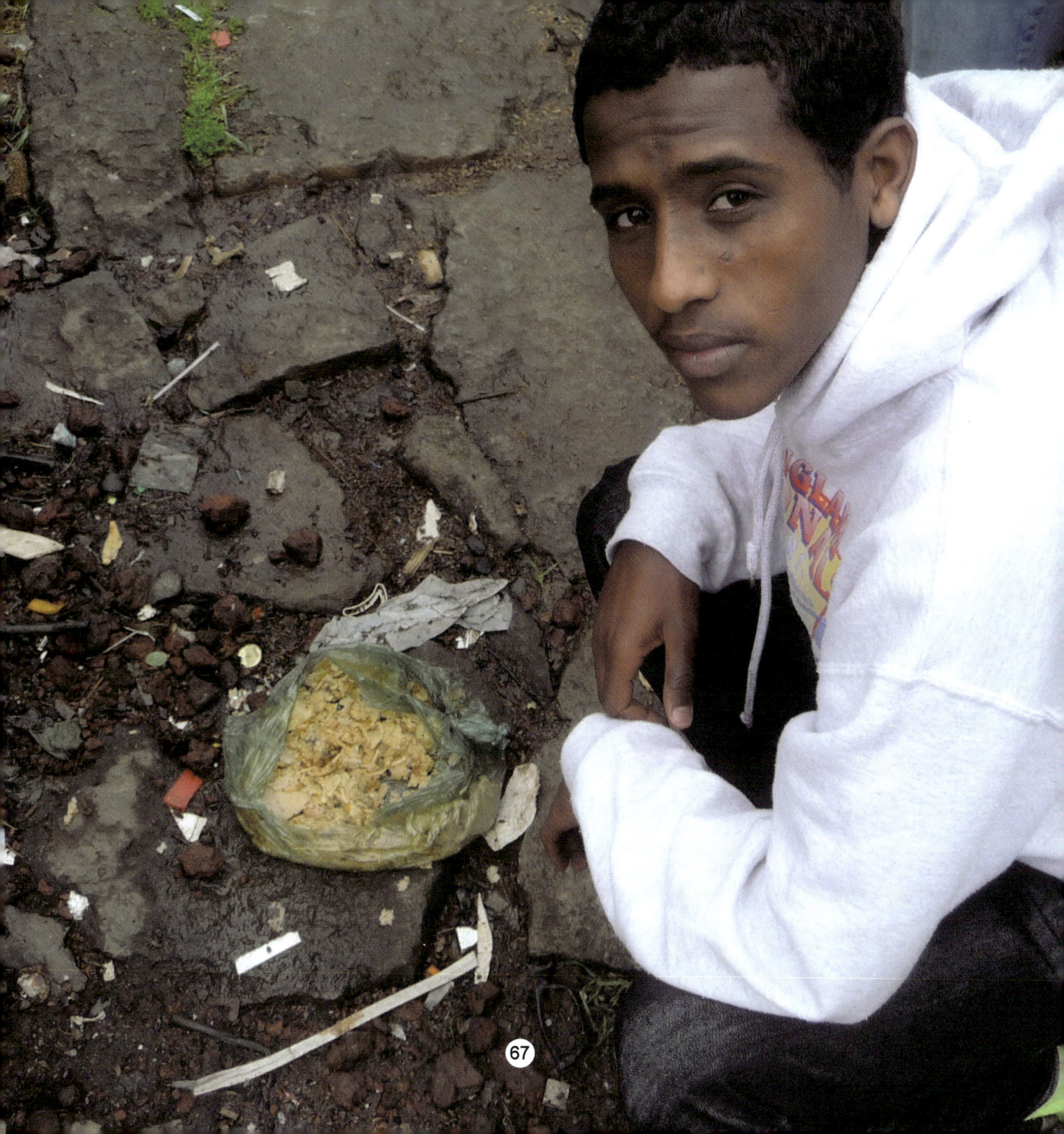

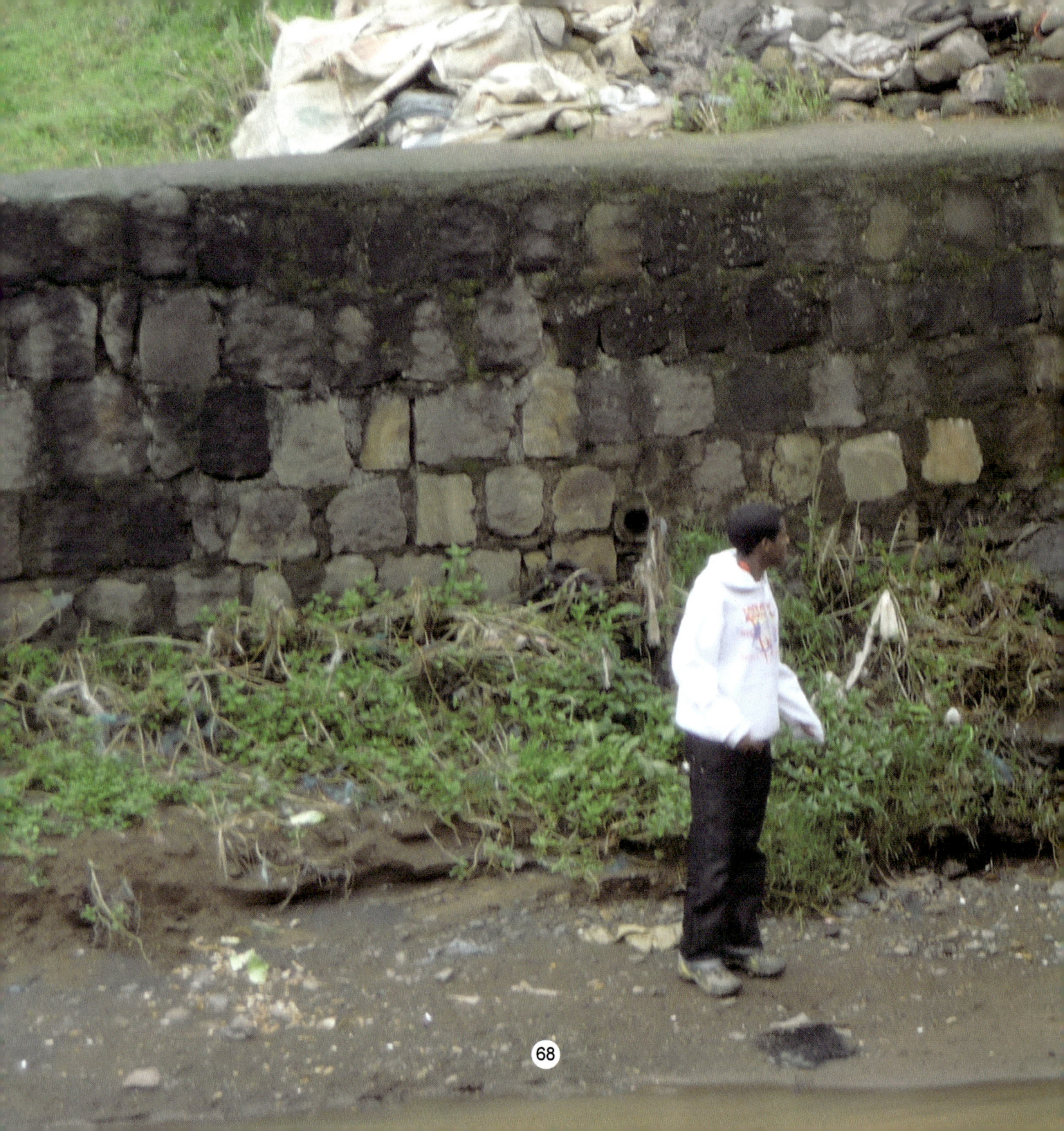

69

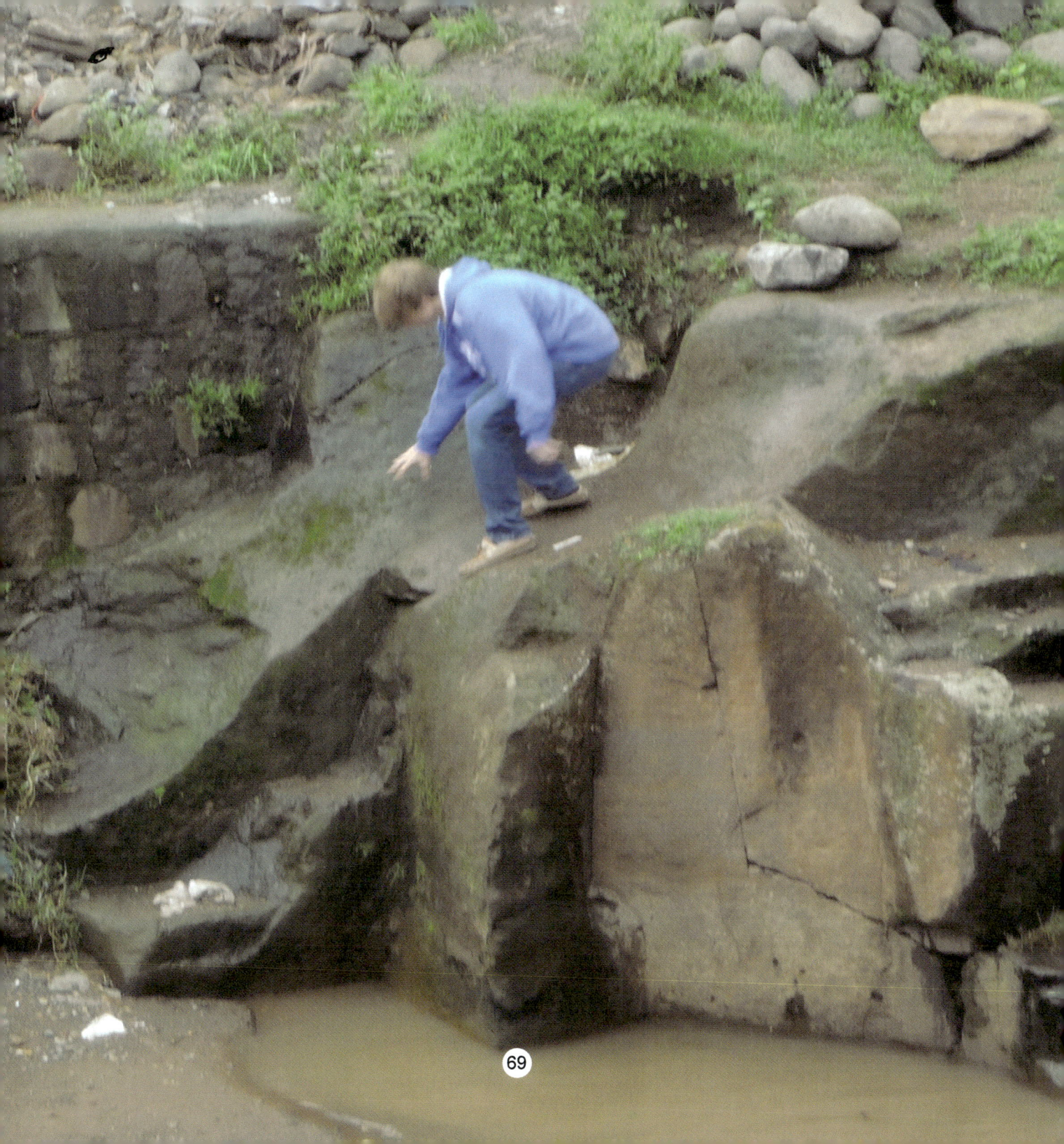

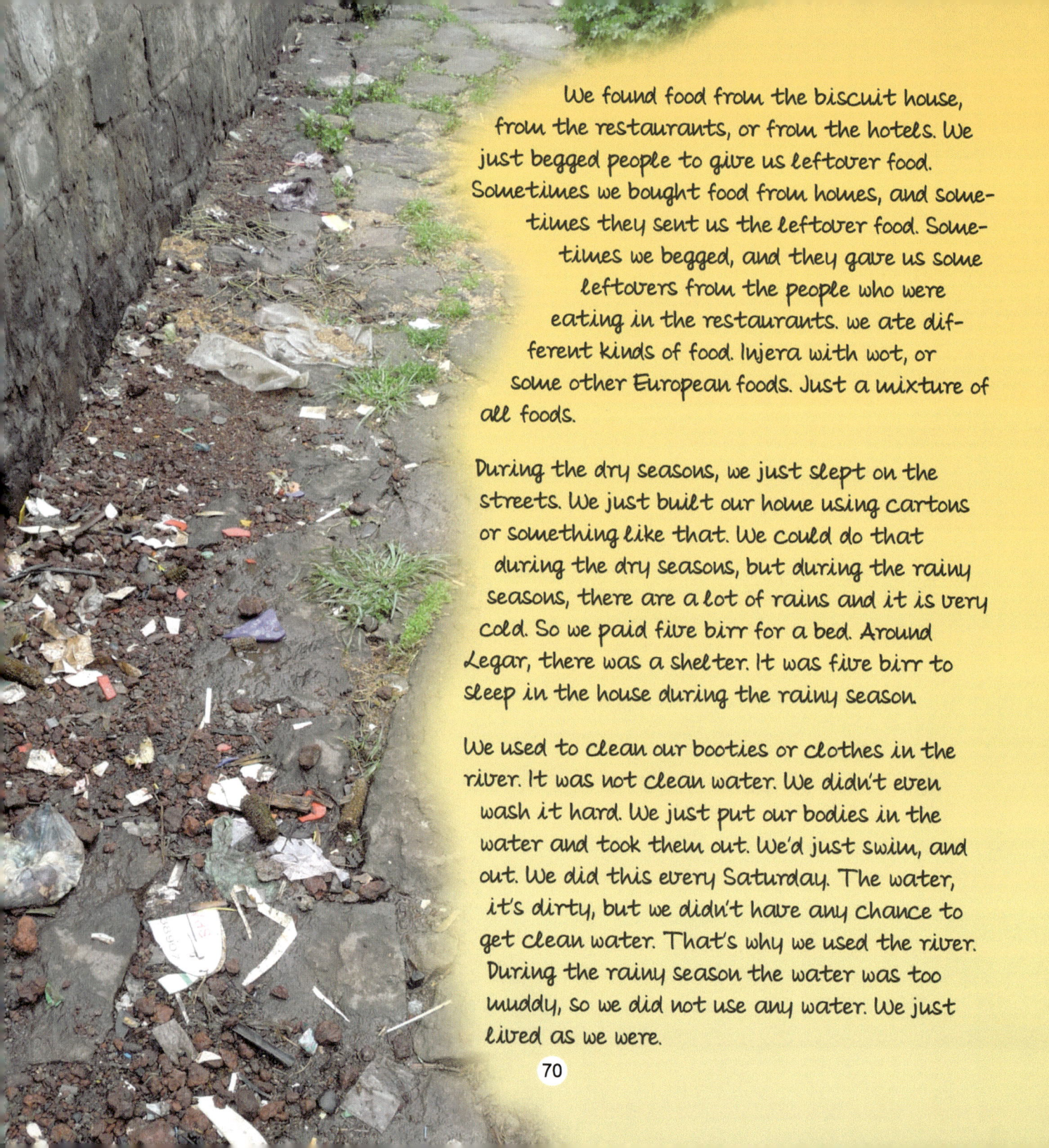

We found food from the biscuit house, from the restaurants, or from the hotels. We just begged people to give us leftover food. Sometimes we bought food from homes, and sometimes they sent us the leftover food. Sometimes we begged, and they gave us some leftovers from the people who were eating in the restaurants. we ate different kinds of food. Injera with wot, or some other European foods. Just a mixture of all foods.

During the dry seasons, we just slept on the streets. We just built our home using cartons or something like that. We could do that during the dry seasons, but during the rainy seasons, there are a lot of rains and it is very cold. So we paid five birr for a bed. Around Legar, there was a shelter. It was five birr to sleep in the house during the rainy season.

We used to clean our booties or clothes in the river. It was not clean water. We didn't even wash it hard. We just put our bodies in the water and took them out. We'd just swim, and out. We did this every Saturday. The water, it's dirty, but we didn't have any chance to get clean water. That's why we used the river. During the rainy season the water was too muddy, so we did not use any water. We just lived as we were.

When we lived on the streets we didn't trust each other. When one person got some money, someone else would be likely to steal the money from him. We learned never to tell anyone how or when we got money, or how much money we had. My friend, Teddy, was the only person I trusted when I was on the streets.

Once, after I worked, I got sixty birr. At the time, sixty birr was big money. Some guys from a gang came to search me and tried to take the money I had earned away from me. I quickly gave it to Teddy, and he ran away. They demanded that I give the money to them, but I didn't have it on me.

Then, after two days, Teddy came back with the sixty birr I had given him. He didn't spend it, not a penny of it. That's how I started to trust him as a friend.

Living on the street is very hard. I watched a friend of mine die. He smoked and chewed a lot, and then he became sick. He got an ulcer and lung cancer. He coughed and coughed. We watched him get sicker and sicker. We took him to the hospital, and they gave him some medicine. Then we brought him back. After two days we found him dead.

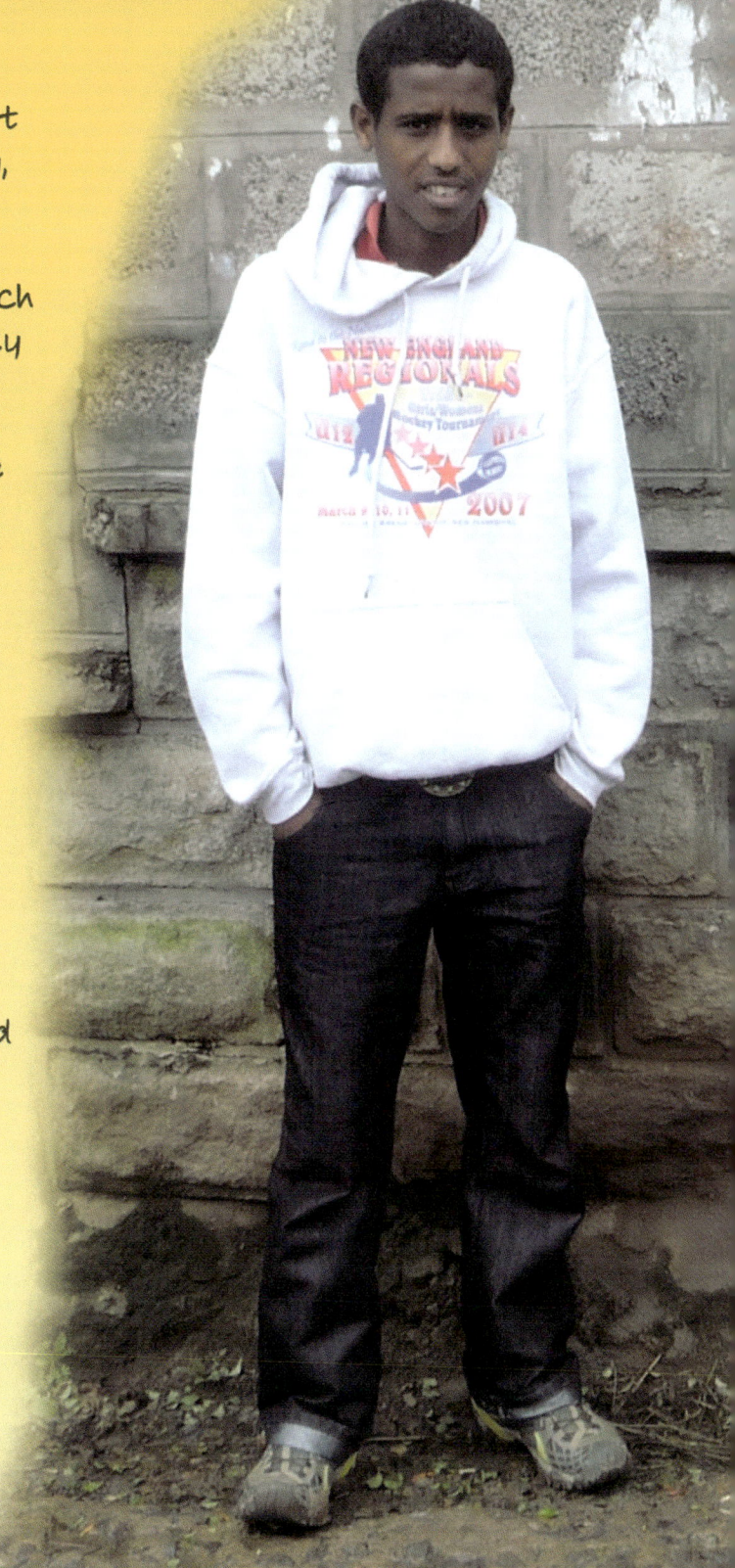

He is still on my mind. When we found him lying there lifeless it was the hardest thing I had ever faced in my life

Then, a little time later, there was also a girl. She had eaten food from restaurants that was spoiled because she was very hungry. We found her dead on the street. Her face color was changed. I started to worry about myself. What would tomorrow bring? I started to think about how I could get out of this. I was afraid.

I don't believe that most of the people wanted to harm us. Sometimes people gave us food and occasionally even money when we begged, but they didn't trust us. They didn't want us too close to them and they didn't want to ask us any questions or talk to them. They just gave us the money and went on their way.

After a while I started feeling empty. After all, if others didn't trust me, what value did I have? When I saw people who were clean or wore a suit, I realized that they saw me as worthless. I started asking myself, "What did I do wrong? What was so wrong for them?" I spent a lot of time thinking about this.

Sometimes boys can protect themselves when they are on the streets, but it is much harder for girls. I saw a lot of girls who faced horrible things. In order to join a group, to be protected by a group, a girl would often have to sell her body. Then she might get pregnant or give birth to a child. Girls faced a lot more problems on the streets than boys did. We might try to help the girls, but we were so young ourselves that we weren't capable of doing much to protect them. The people who hurt the girls were older than we were. It was very difficult for us to help the girls because we were children ourselves.

Sometimes the girls and the boys would get drunk together. They would come back to the place where we slept and have sex. Many times I saw this. It wasn't by force except by the force of alcohol.

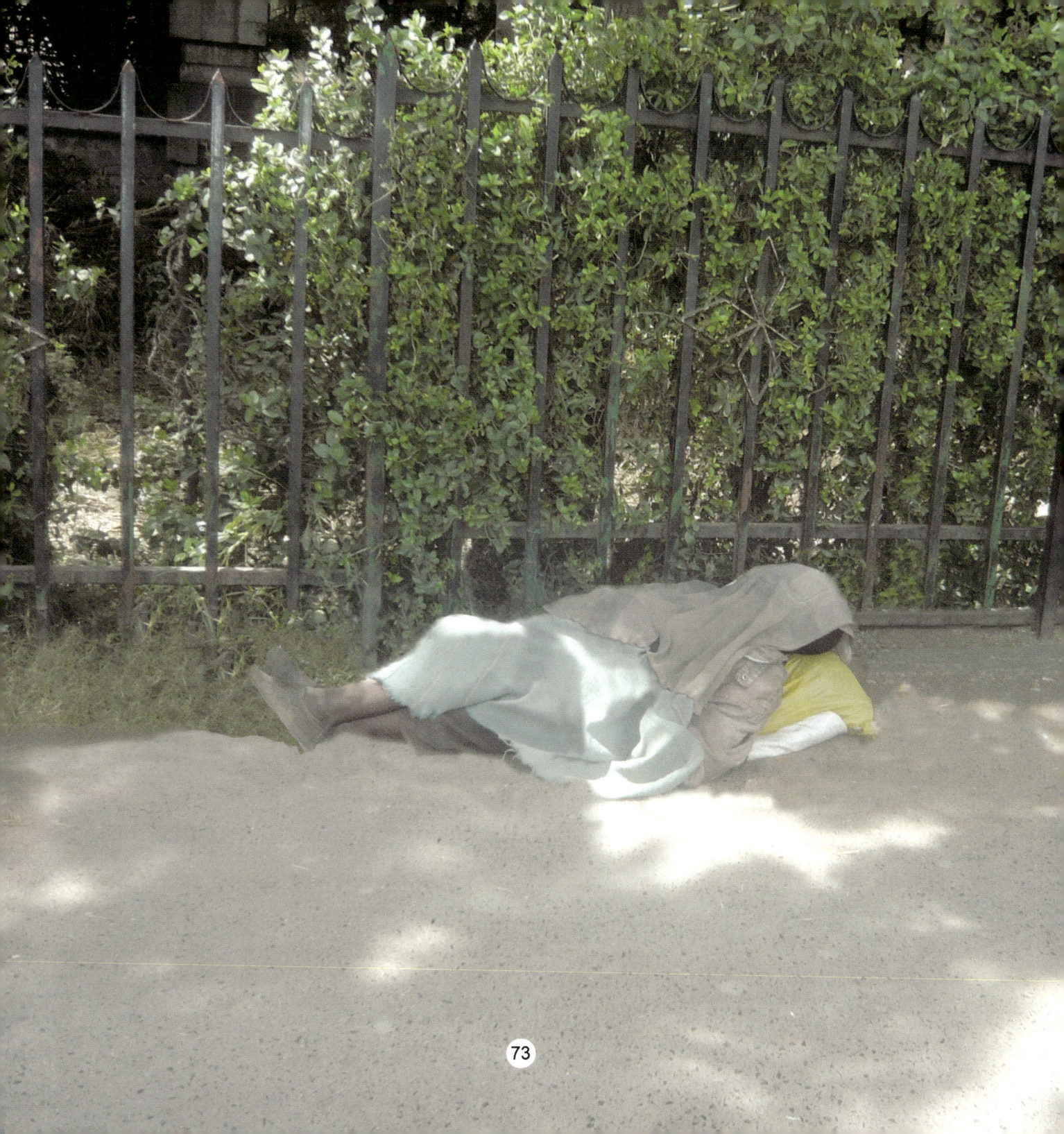

Several years ago many of the street children were taken to jail. That was one of the most frightening times I can remember. I never understood the reason why they took only the street children to jail. We actually escaped, but I don't know how.

A friend of mine was put in jail, and then they just released him after a time. He told us how very difficult it was to survive in the jail. He was taken to a very deserted area, and they got bread only once a day. The wardens cut his hair.

Having my friend, Teddy, beside me was my best hope for survival. One of the things that gave me the confidence to try to escape from that life was my belief that I had a talent that would help me, and that was music. Sometimes I was even hired in a club that worked to prevent HIV. So I had hope.

When I was a child in the countryside, I used to sing when I was alone. Now that singing has developed into a true love for music. I get a lot of my satisfaction from music.

When I was living on the streets, I always appreciated people who wanted to help me, or other street children like me. I also appreciated any singers. I loved listening to music. And I really appreciated the person who gave us that bread and tea at Hope Enterprise. He was very kind to us.

My faith played a strong role in helping me to change my life. I believe, or I trusted in God. I even stayed overnight at the churches sometimes, and I always prayed for God to help me. I believe that's why I am not addicted to drugs or something like that now. That is how I got to Selamta. God helped me. We would go to church, but not every day. I don't have a way to describe God. It's beyond my scope, I think, but I know that he has helped me a lot.

I believe that it is God who created the Earth and he gave us everything. He gave us two choices: bad or good. It's up to us to choose which one we will take.

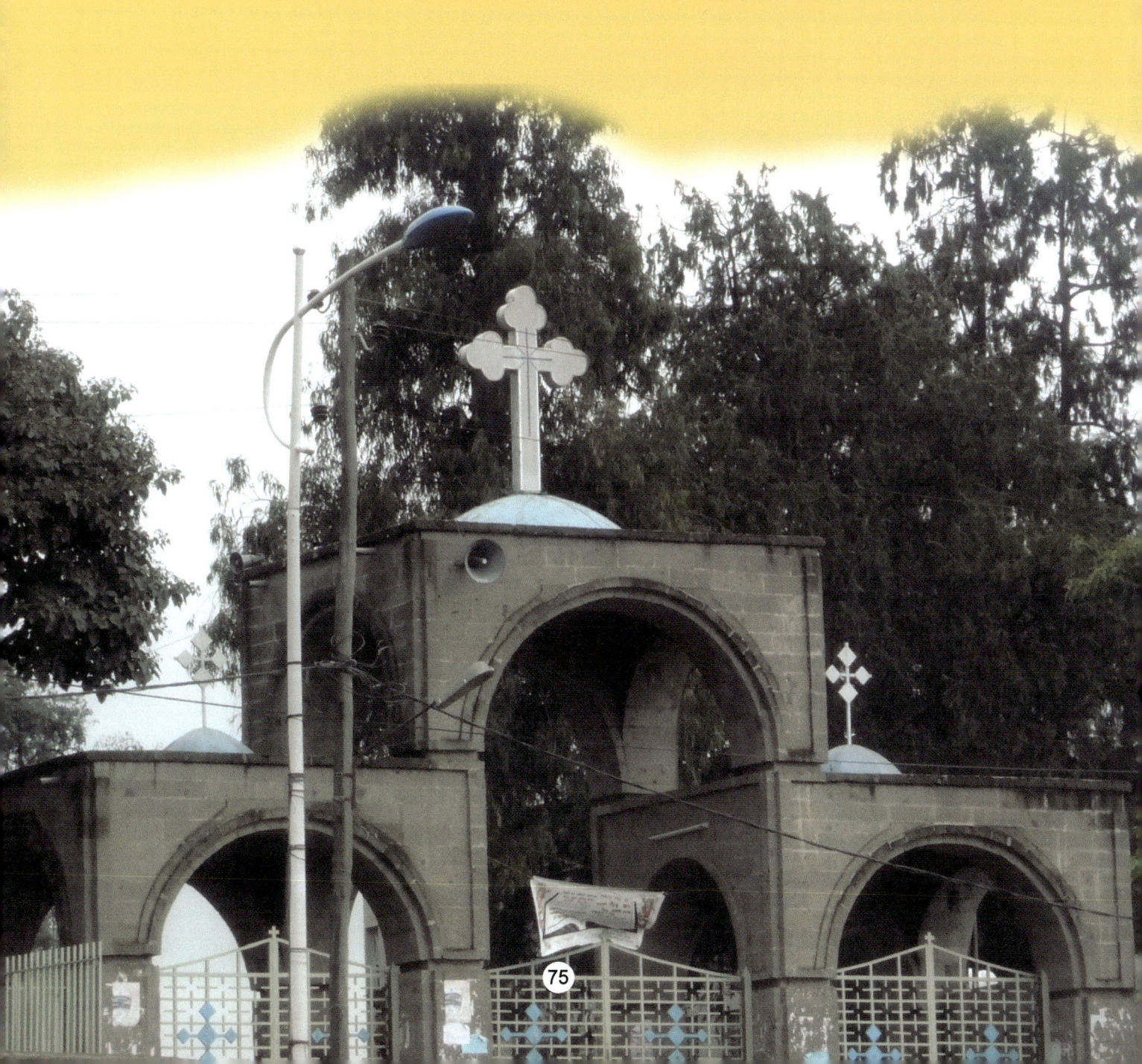

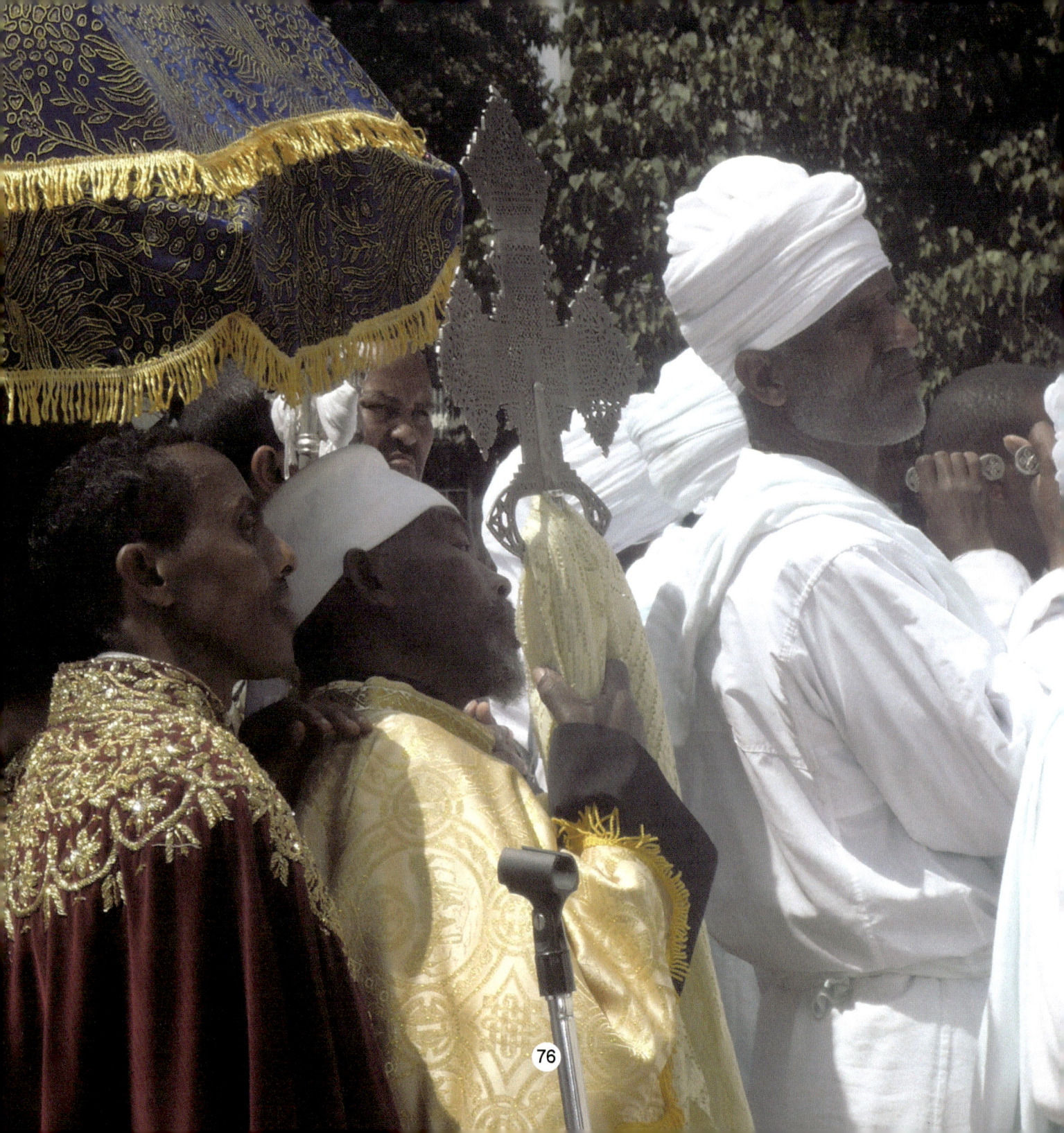

77

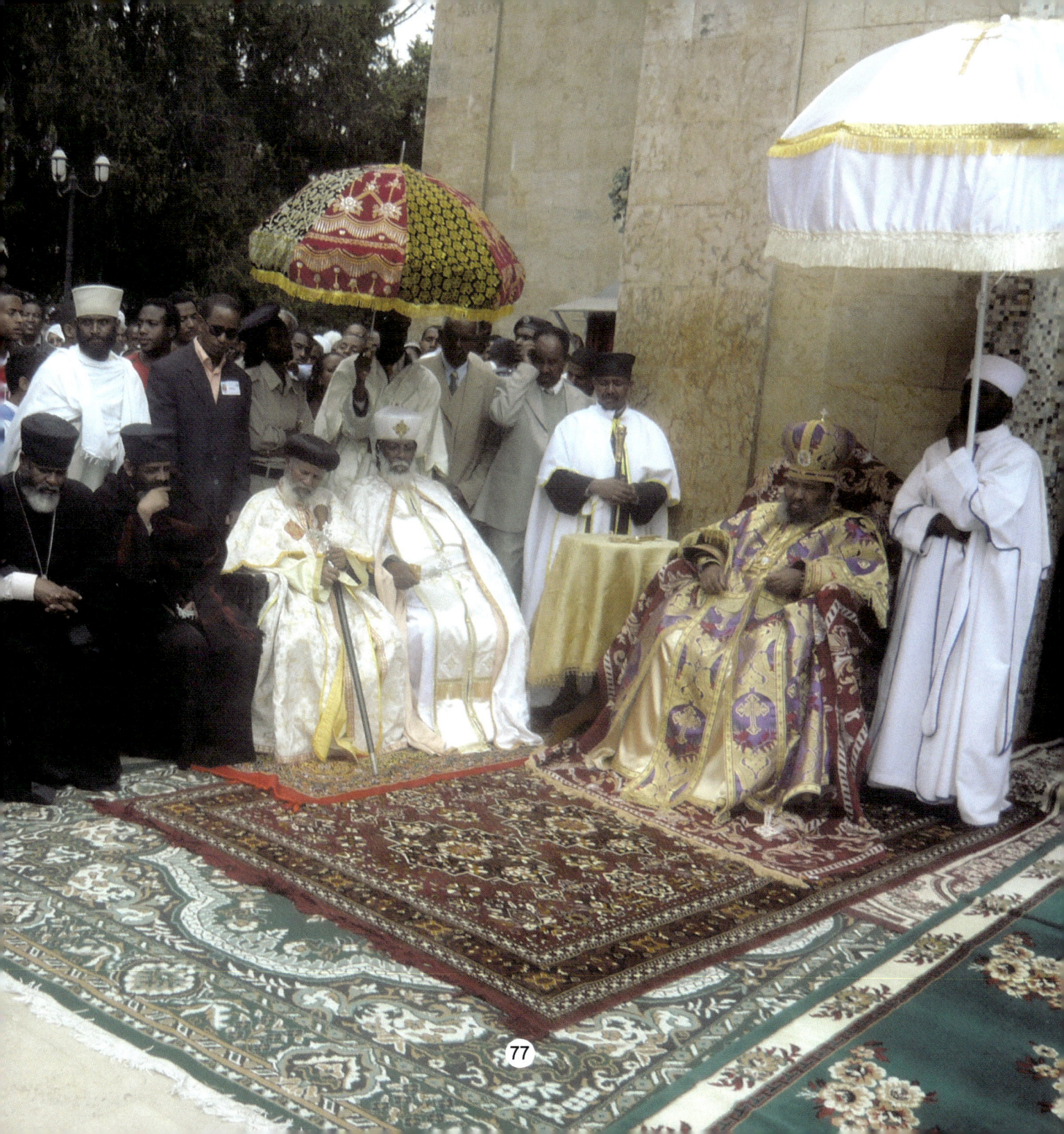

A Special Dinner

Chris:

Some days we just spent time with the children reading books and discussing values and life skills. The kids seem to soak up any information they have access to, and clearly have an innate desire to please other people, do well, and receive praise.

One night, I had a special surprise planned for dinner for Robel and his family. Esmael came to pick us up, and we went out to eat at a traditional Ethiopian style restaurant. There was dancing, singing and music throughout the restaurant. It was the first time that the family had been together to a restaurant, and they clearly loved it. I was surprised to see how much even the smallest child could eat! Robel's mother and the children sat mesmerized at the live dancers and performing artists. The nonstop dancing and singing definitely delighted them. I was happy that I could be a part of their first night out to a restaurant.

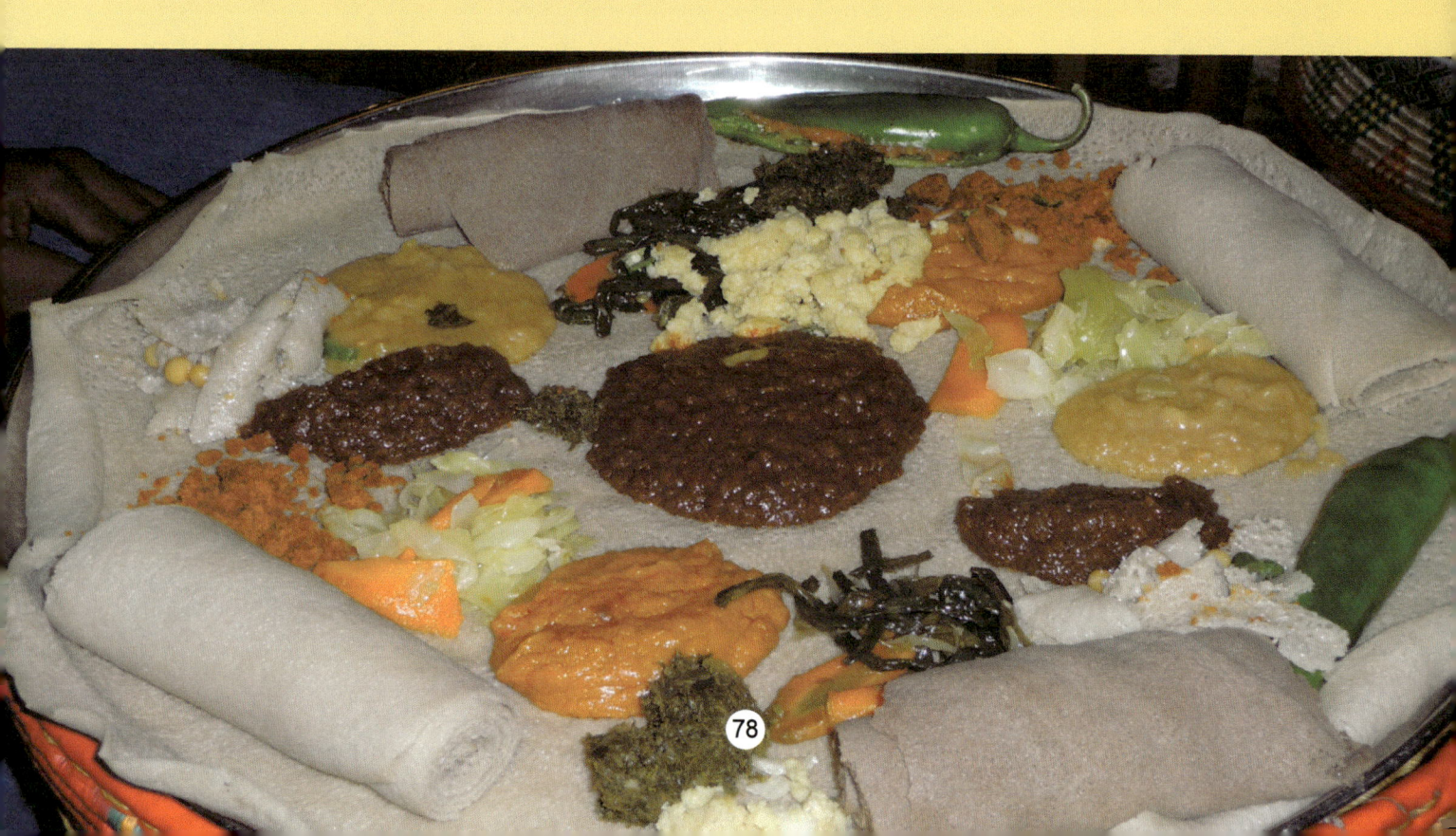

79

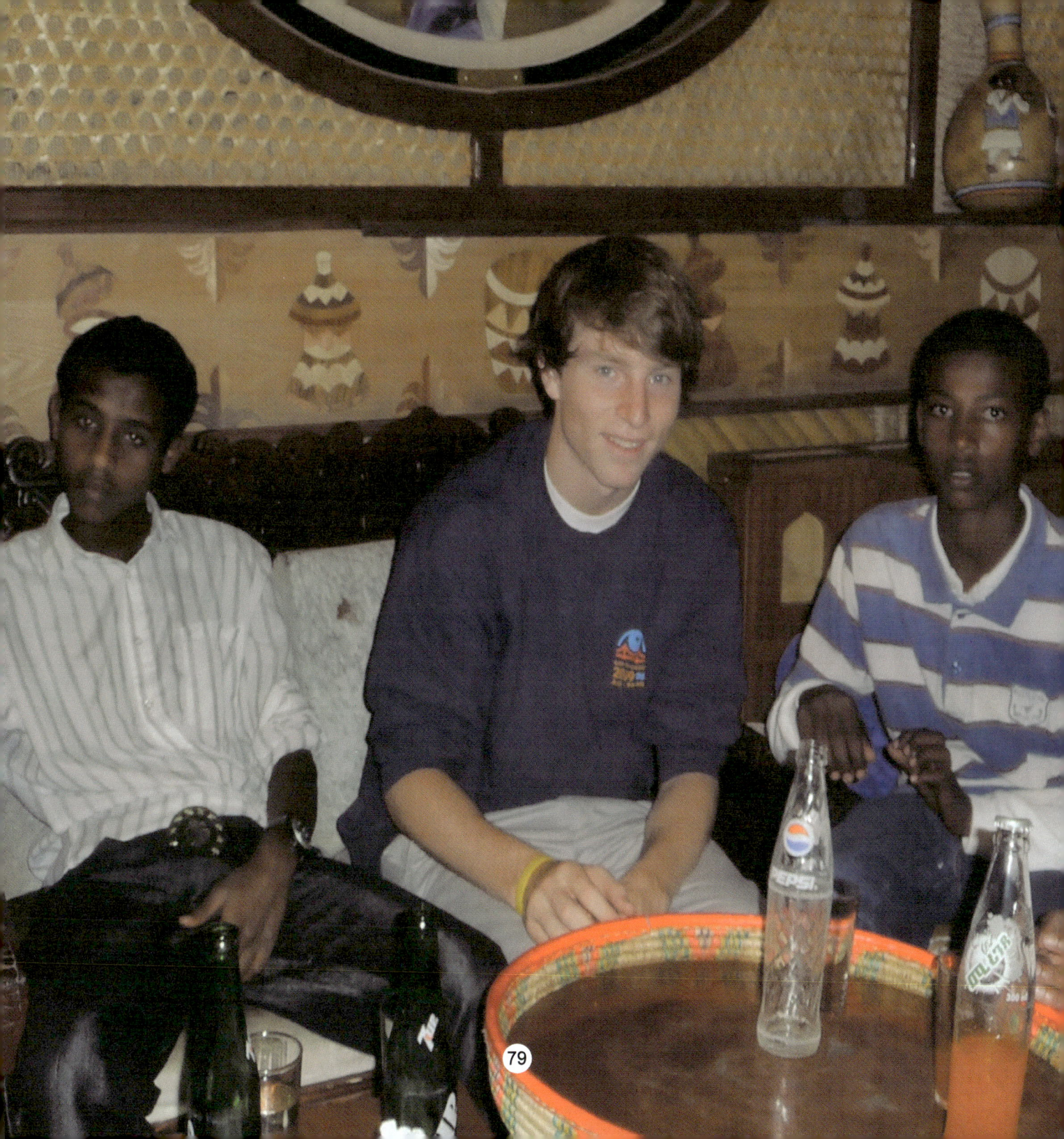

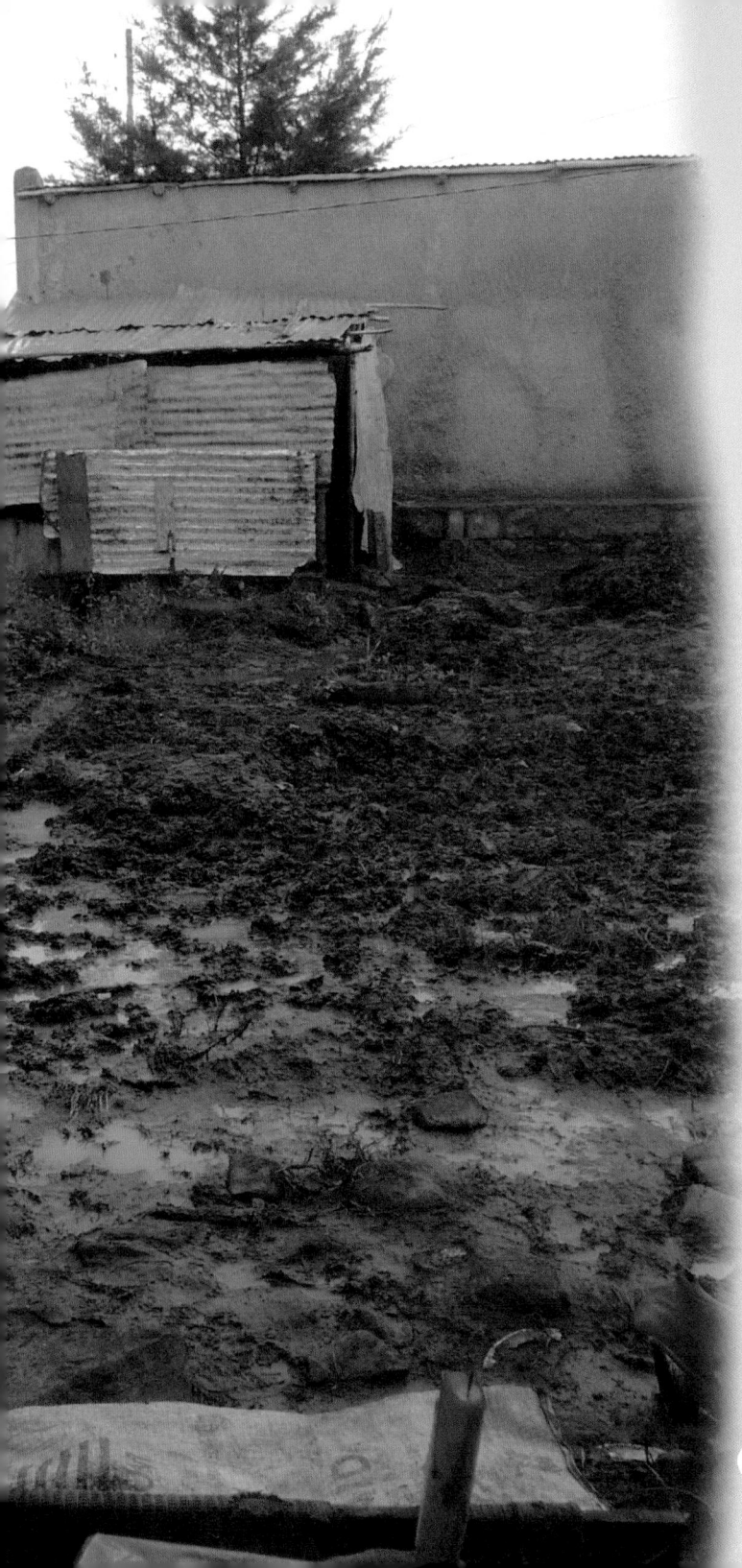

Mekdes and Yeshi

Chris:

Most of the Selamta families are within a mile of each other in the town of Bethel, a suburb of Addis Ababa. But Selamta also supports some children living in their own homes outside of the immediate area. These kids are part of the outreach program. The outreach program is designed to provide money to certain people who Selamta has been connected with through the Ethiopian government. They are not a part of Selamta families, but get some support from the program. One day we took the new van and traveled to the suburbs of Addis to visit one of these families.

As the new van approached the outreach house, traveling down an unpaved road full of potholes and animals, I kept thinking that in America this would be called a "slum." This "family" consisted of two girls, Mekdes, who is seventeen years old and Yeshi, who is twelve years old. No one from Selamta had ever visited these girls because of the long distance from Selamta. As we approached, the girls opened the tin door of their home- one room, made of dirt, straw and cow manure supporting a tin roof riddled with holes.

I thought that they just looked like little kids, standing there at the door smiling at strangers. Their front yard was mud and manure, with polluted water pooled between the piles. I wondered how anyone could survive in such dire circumstances. Here were two young girls living all alone in a hovel, with only the love between them keeping them together and hopeful.

Medkes prepared traditional Ethiopian coffee for us-clearly she was a kind and considerate girl. Medkes explained that she had no recollection of her father, and that her mother had died over four years ago. She and her sister watched their mother commit suicide by an overdose of medication that she believed to have been used to alleviate the pain from AIDS.

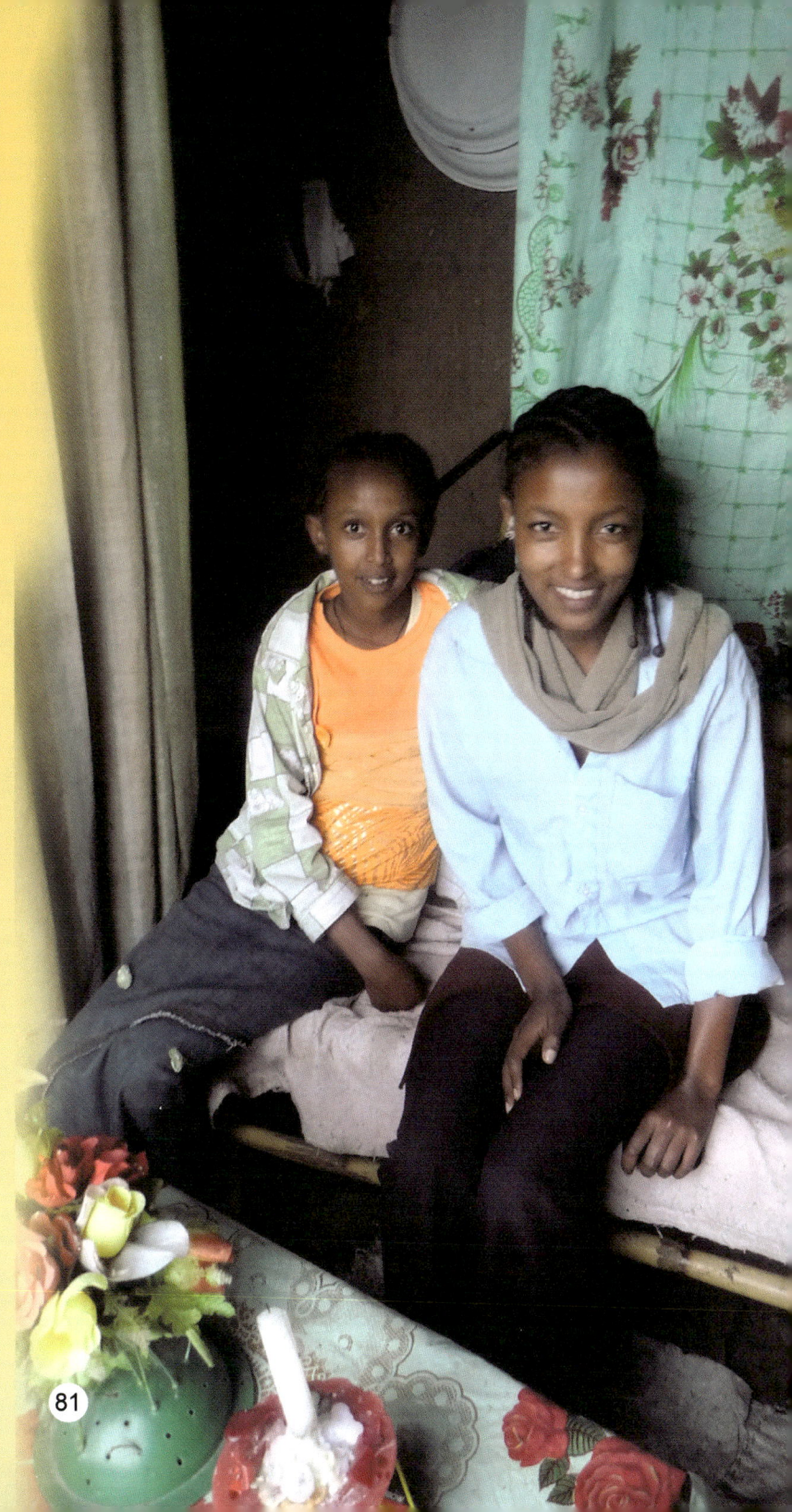

After their mother died, they had stayed in their house, and Medkes had been working in a cotton factory for 8 Birr ($.50) a day, in an effort to improve the living situation for her and her sister. Recently, due to the fact that these jobs were scarce, she was laid off from her work. Their only source of income was the Selamta Outreach family. She told me that without the Selamta support, they would be on the streets; she was happy to have that leaky tin roof over their heads. More than anything, these two sisters wanted to be with each other.

Medkes had spent what in America would have been her middle school years, being the parent to her younger sister. From what I could tell, she had done a great job. Yeshi was polite, listened attentively to her sister, and every once in a while I noticed that she would glance at us. Both girls attended private schools, using the money from the Outreach program, and each girl loved school and learning. At night, they would study and read for hours, and I suspect hope that maybe the next day their lives would be a little easier.

As we were getting ready to leave them to return to Selamta, I noticed some white cloth with a yarn string in Medkes ear, and I asked her about it. She said that intermittently her ear would ache and leak white liquid, and that this had been happening since her mother had died. I was shocked!.

For over four years, she had an untreated ear infection, and nothing had been done about it. I immediately gave her all the money I had with me, and asked her to please use it to go to the doctor and get treatment. A medical check up is 50 birr and for an additional 150-200 Birr, she could obtain antibiotics. In total, I gave her less than $50 US, which I was told, was plenty.

I was appalled that for more than four years she had a constant ear problem and nothing had been done. She had been working for her family, studying in school and did not have the time or money to seek medical assistance. When I got back to Selamta that night, I hoped and prayed that I had given her enough money so that she could finally get treatment. And most of all, I hoped and prayed that those two young girls could come and live within Selamta.

83

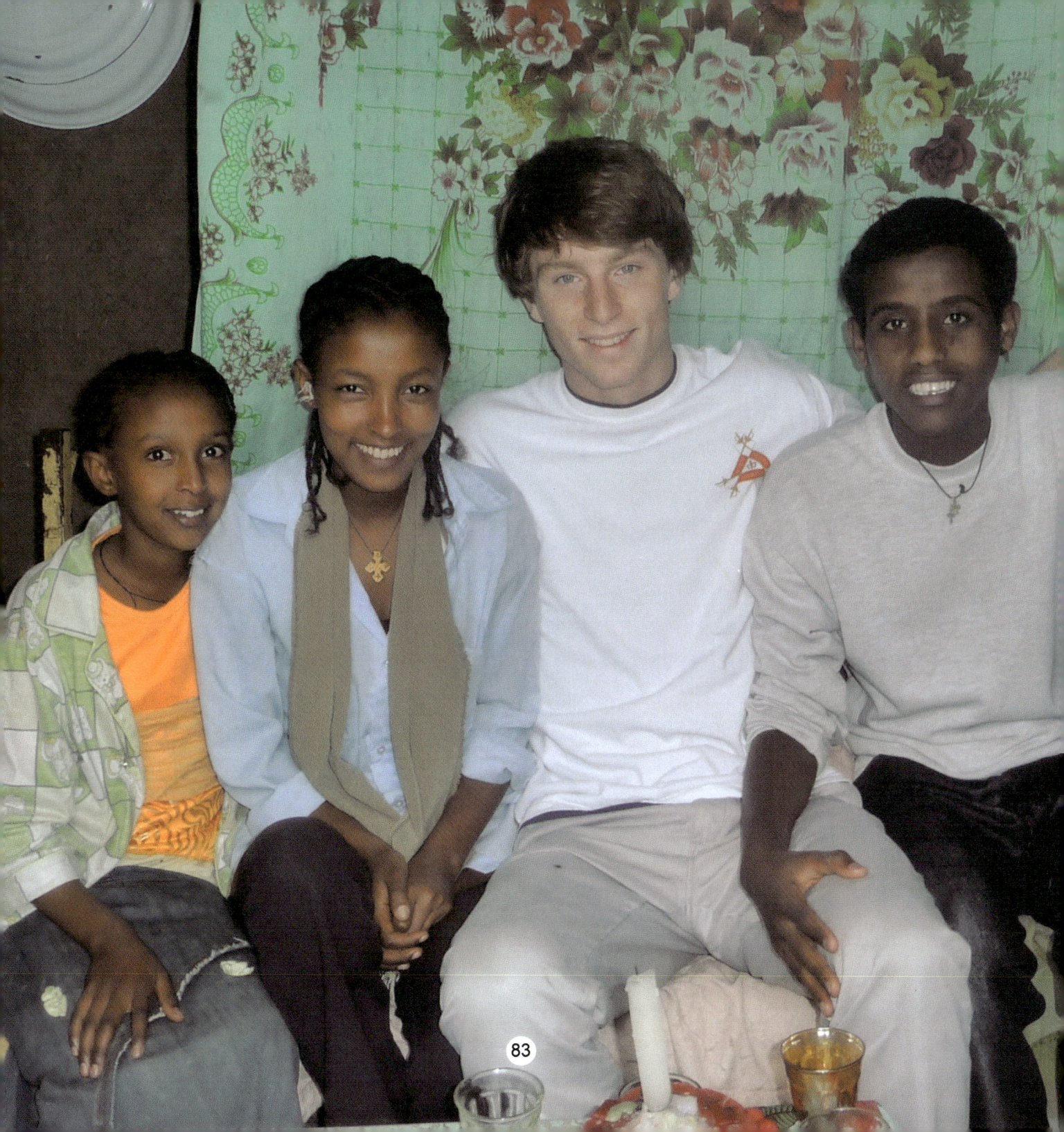

Robel:

When I saw the way Yeshi and Mekdes were living, I had a bad feeling. I worried about their health and whether they were getting enough food to eat. We thought they would be happier and better cared for if they moved into one of the Selamta families, so we worked to get them to join Selamta. I don't believe that they have enough money to survive with only 800 birr per month (less than $77), for both of them. It would be better for them to come to Selamta. That was my feeling.

*****

Now I am so happy to say that they are here with us at Selamta. I asked them, after they had been here for three or four days, how their life changed. They thought about he difference between their lives here and the way their lives were outside, and they smiled and said, "It's very nice here!"

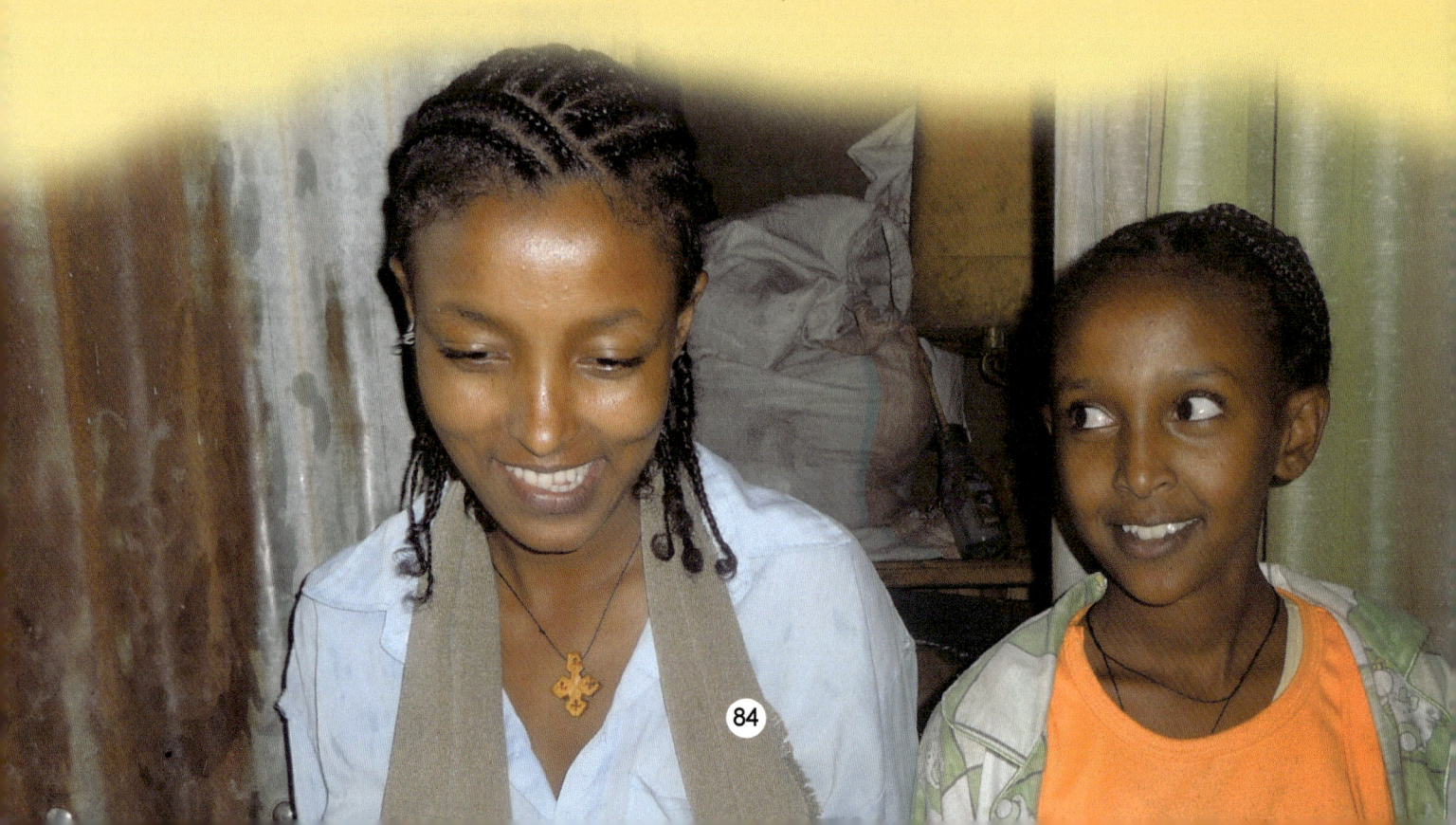

85

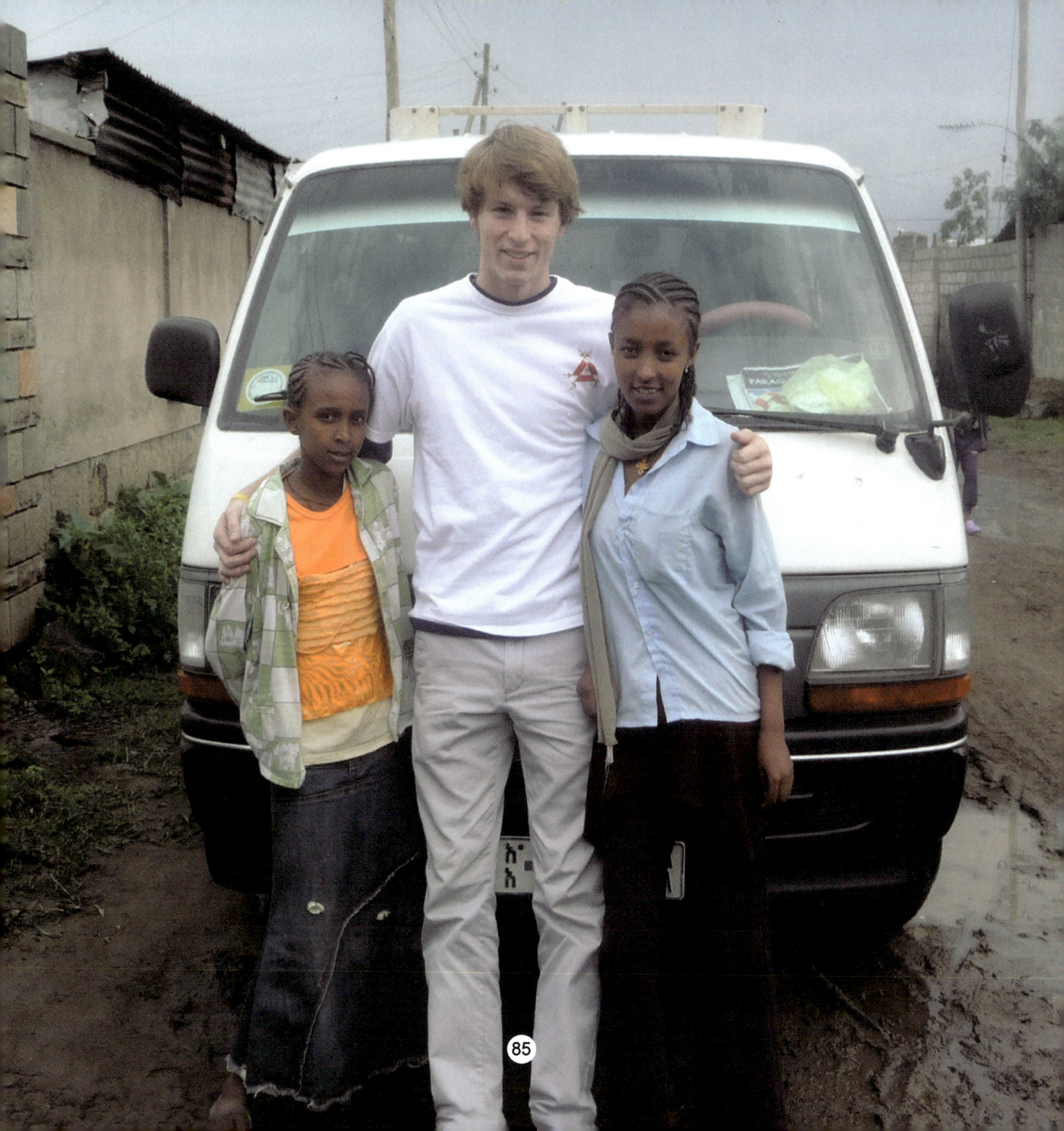

Chris:

The rest of my time in Ethiopia was spent with Robel and the other children of Selamta, working and playing. When it was time for me to return to the United States, I didn't want to leave. Even the smallest gesture is appreciated by the children of Selamta. These children have overcome seemingly insurmountable obstacles, yet each has learned to love and trust within a new family.

Leaving Robel was particularly difficult, as I have come to think of him as a brother. I have such admiration for him and the sheer will and determination that that he has employed to made his own life better. Robel has overcome extraordinary challenges, and his story is one of hope and survival. To have seen first-hand the streets where Robel lived for years, to hear his story of loss and survival, and to experience it through him makes me have tremendous respect and love for him. Robel recognizes and appreciates the opportunities given to him by the Selamta Family Project, and serves as an example of a bright future for Ethiopia.

Robel:

Chris came over here to visit me, and we shared a great deal together. He has talked with me about a lot of things. He taught me things and helped me. I appreciate that very much. I was happy I could show him some history and culture of Ethiopia to go with some of the difficult things we face. And If I ever have a chance to go to the US to visit Chris in his hometown, I'd be very happy.

I will always pray: God make me a friend or a brother with Chris. Keep us the best of friends.

87

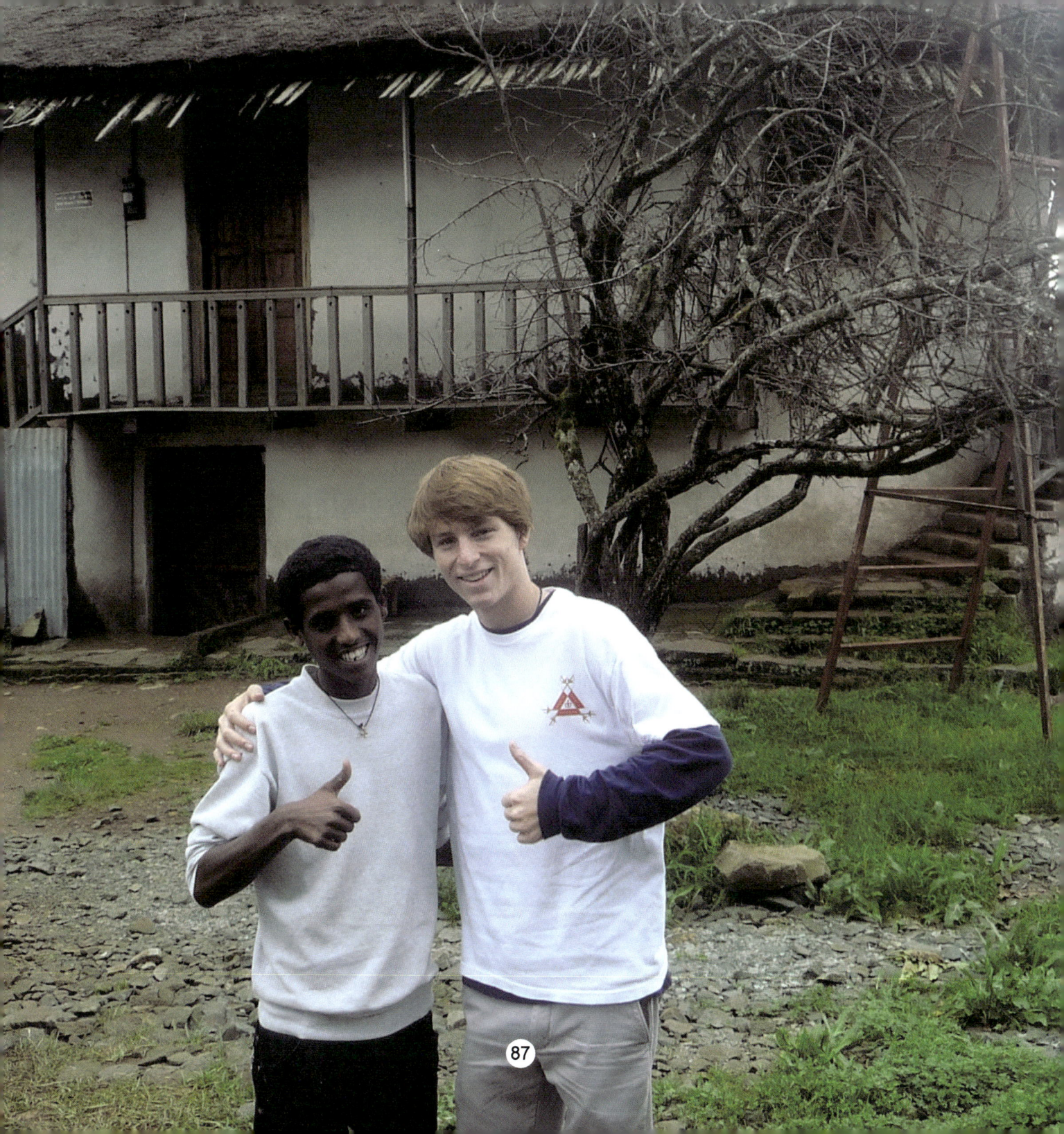

Afterword

Chris:

I have settled back into my comfortable life in the United States. I have kept in touch with my Selamta friends, and am happy that they continue to work hard and find success.

Robel continues to practice his music, and improves on a daily basis. Robel's last letter said, "For me a friend is just like a brother who shares a lot of things with you. You are even more than a friend. Even though we have different skin, we are just brothers. I will always pray: God keep me as a friend or a brother with you. Make us the best of friends." Robel wanted me to share with my American friends that the children of Selamta are "open-minded and quick learners. If they get the chance, they are ready to change themselves." Robel should know, and he is right.

I also received notice that after I shared the housing conditions of Yeshi and Mekdes Chernet, the Outreach children, they were brought to live in Selamta. I am their American sponsor, and I received a letter from them thanking me for helping to get them to Selamta. Their most recent letter ended with, "wishing you all the best things in life, until we meet again." I know that time will come.

Selamta: "Be at Peace."

89

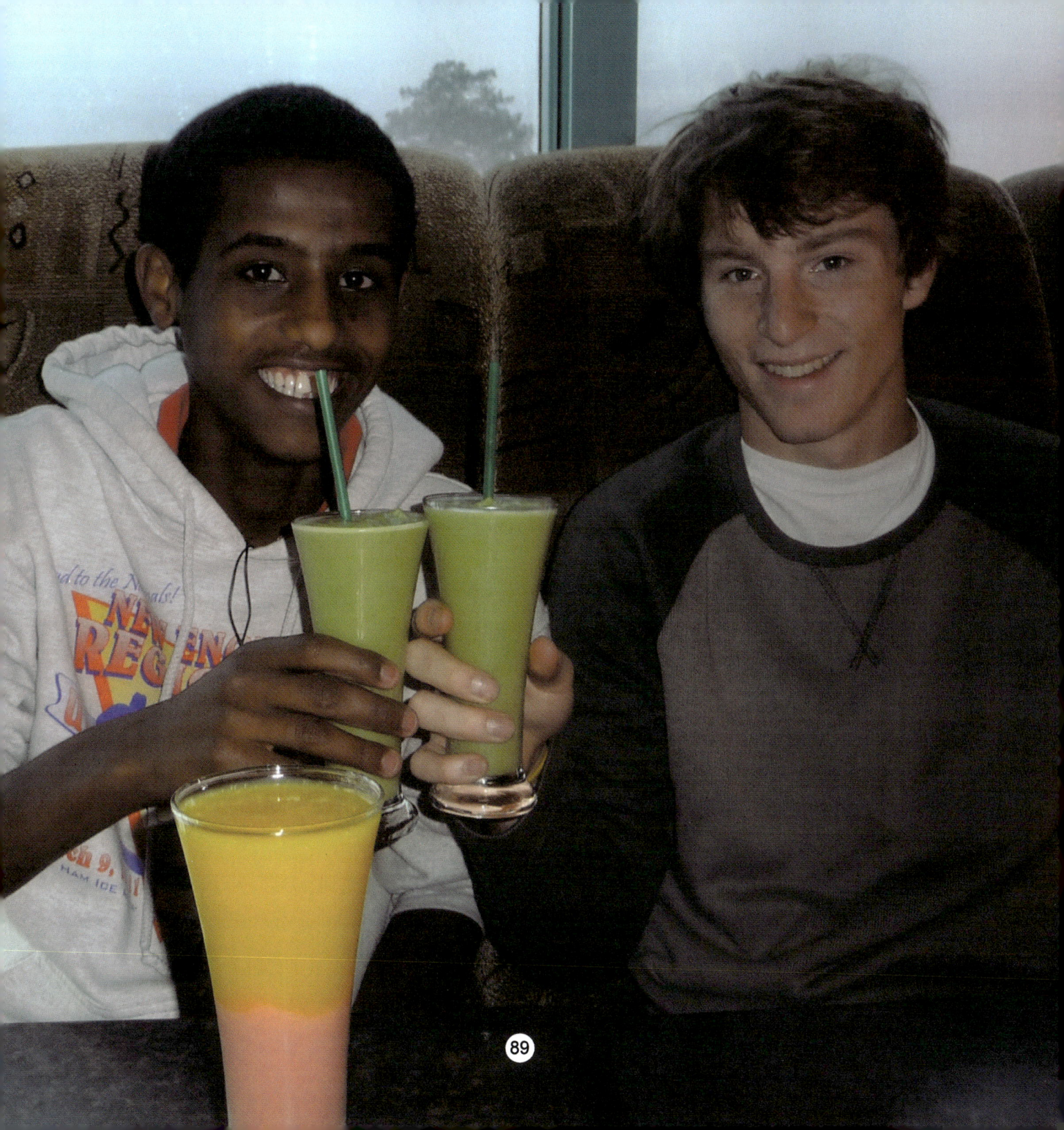

90

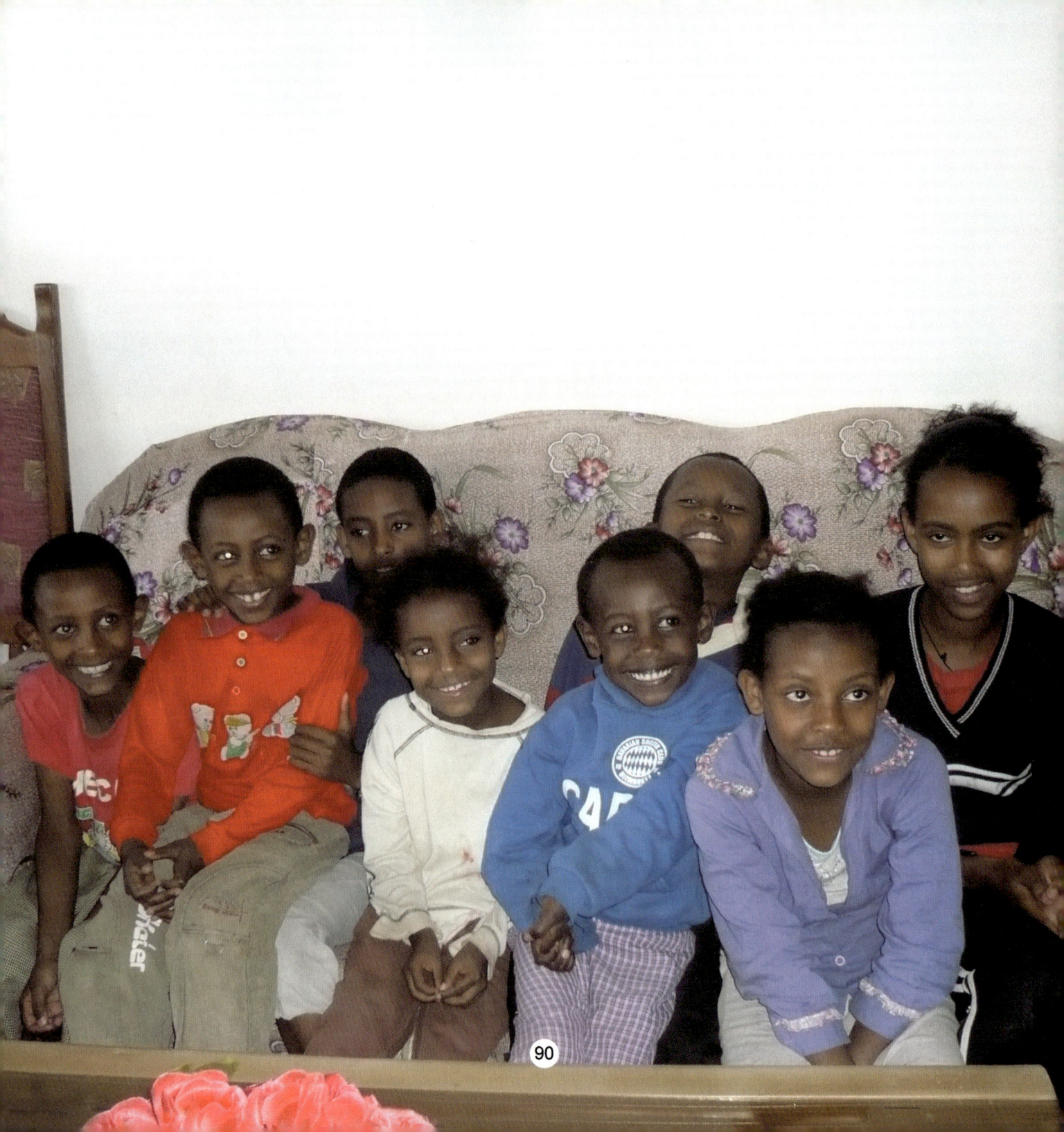

SELAMTA
FAMILY PROJECT

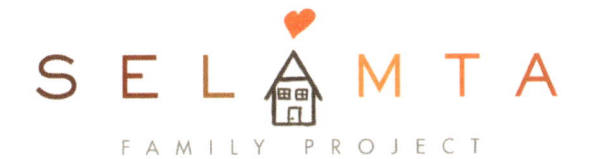

THE CRISIS

More than four million children in Ethiopia have been orphaned by AIDS in a country with no societal safety net. The overwhelming majority are separated from their siblings and abandoned to the streets. Some are placed in orphanages where they routinely encounter violence, predation or abuse. These children are joined in poverty by millions of displaced women who have lost their adult children and husbands to AIDS.

THE SOLUTION

The Selamta Project creates new, stable, and life-long families for children to repair the social fabric of their society. For the past six years, we have tested the power of a formula that takes children from the streets, reunites them with lost siblings, stabilizes them emotionally, and creates a new family around them. In the process, we have established new family homes in a constellation around a center that serves newly arriving children and the community at large.

Children simply deserve room to grow in a predictable home, supported with proper nutrition, health care, education and love. The Selamta Project is proving that these objectives are not beyond our reach. Selamta is a unique and successful model, and our mission is to grow into a platform for positive change throughout Ethiopia, Africa and beyond.

Why is Selamta different? Selamta doesn't help orphans: it creates families. According to Unicef and other leading organizations for children, stable families are the most successful model for social change and renewal.

Here's what makes Selamta unique:
• Every Selamta family comprises a mother, an "auntie", and up to 9 siblings ranging in age from infants to young adults. Some children are biological siblings; others become siblings. All are fiercely loyal brothers and sisters, and share remarkably strong bonds of love and commitment.

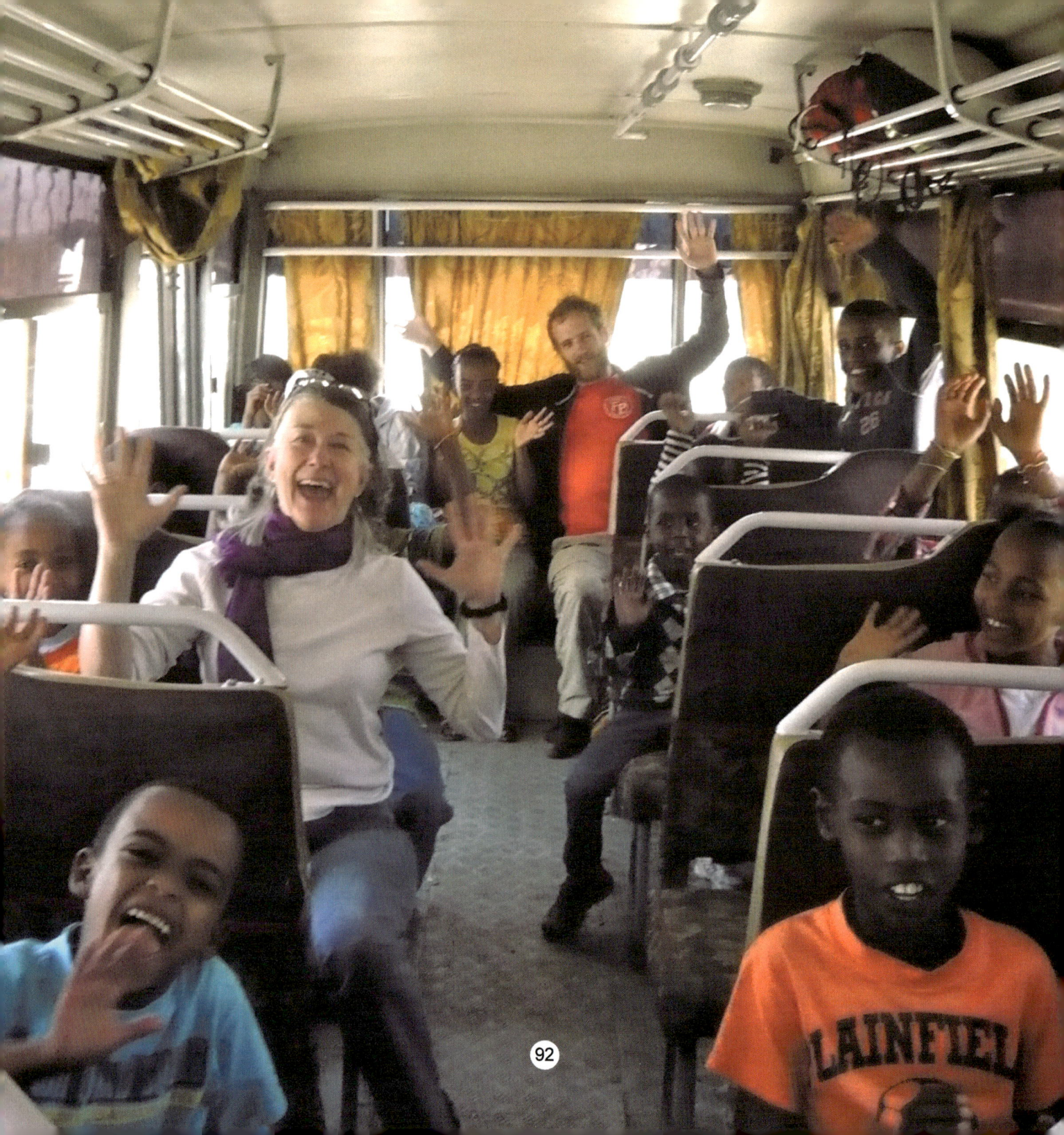

- Selamta families accept older children and large sibling groups. We work to reunite siblings who have been separated and bring them together.

- The women of Selamta have created a strong peer-to-peer support network and meet at least once a week. The mothers and aunties of Selamta are women who have been marginalized by society. They receive training to help them succeed at parenting and running a household and attend ongoing workshops that cover topics ranging from issues specific to orphan care such as trauma, loss, and signs of depression to parenting, nutrition, and budgeting.

- Half of the youth at Selamta are female and we encourage them to be leaders in their community. Our girls are members of the Selamta Parliament, a group of youth, moms, & staff who meet to discuss various matters concerning Selamta.
At the close of last school year 17 of our girls ranked among the top 10 students in their individual class.

- No one "ages out" at Selamta. Selamta families are not temporary fixes. Rather, they are life-long families and will remain so even as the children of Selamta become adults and raise families of their own.

- Selamta families keep Ethiopian children in their own culture, strengthening the fabric of their communities. Each Selamta family is well integrated in their neighborhood, and the stigma of AIDS is falling away as friends and neighbors realize these are families like any other.

- Selamta provides its families with HIV/AIDS prevention education to prevent the spread of HIV/AIDS in future generations.

- Selamta includes an outreach program, designed to support families in the community who are caring for children who have lost parents. The Selamta model recognizes that maintaining primary family ties is the best solution for children who have been orphaned.

For more information see http://www.selamtafamilyproject.org

94

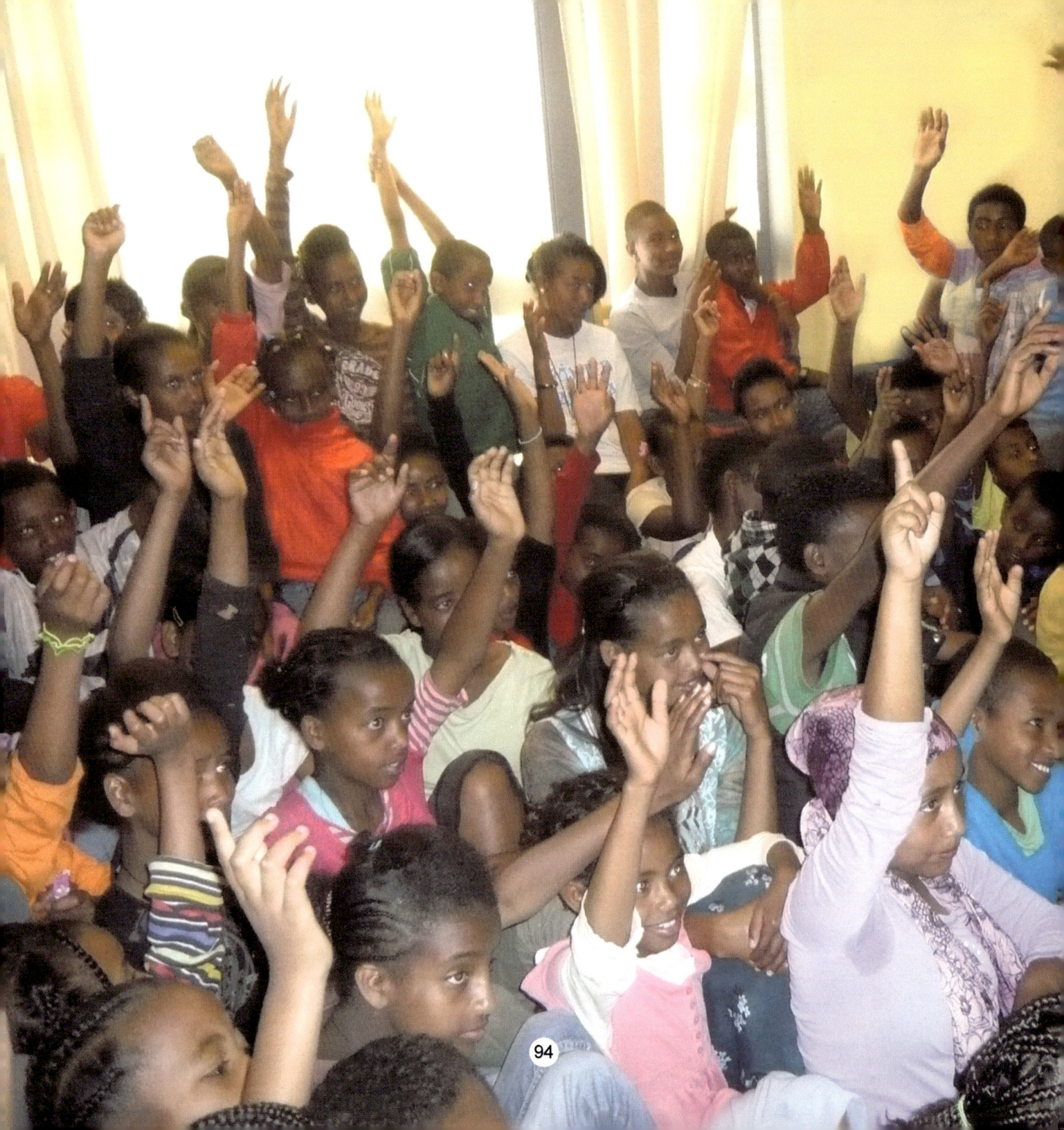

95

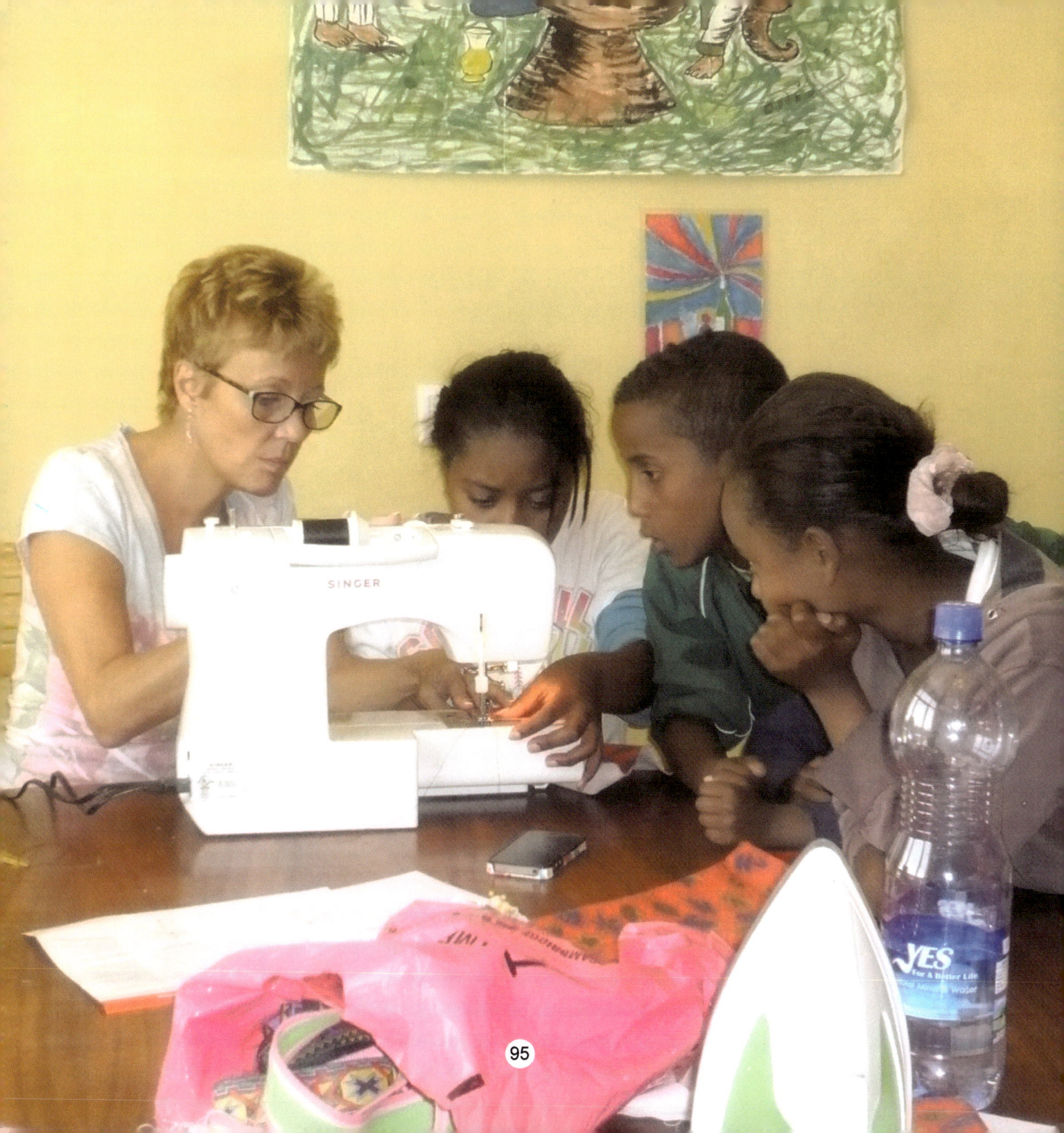

"Never underestimate the power of a small group of committed people to change the world. In fact, it is the only thing that ever has."

Margaret Mead

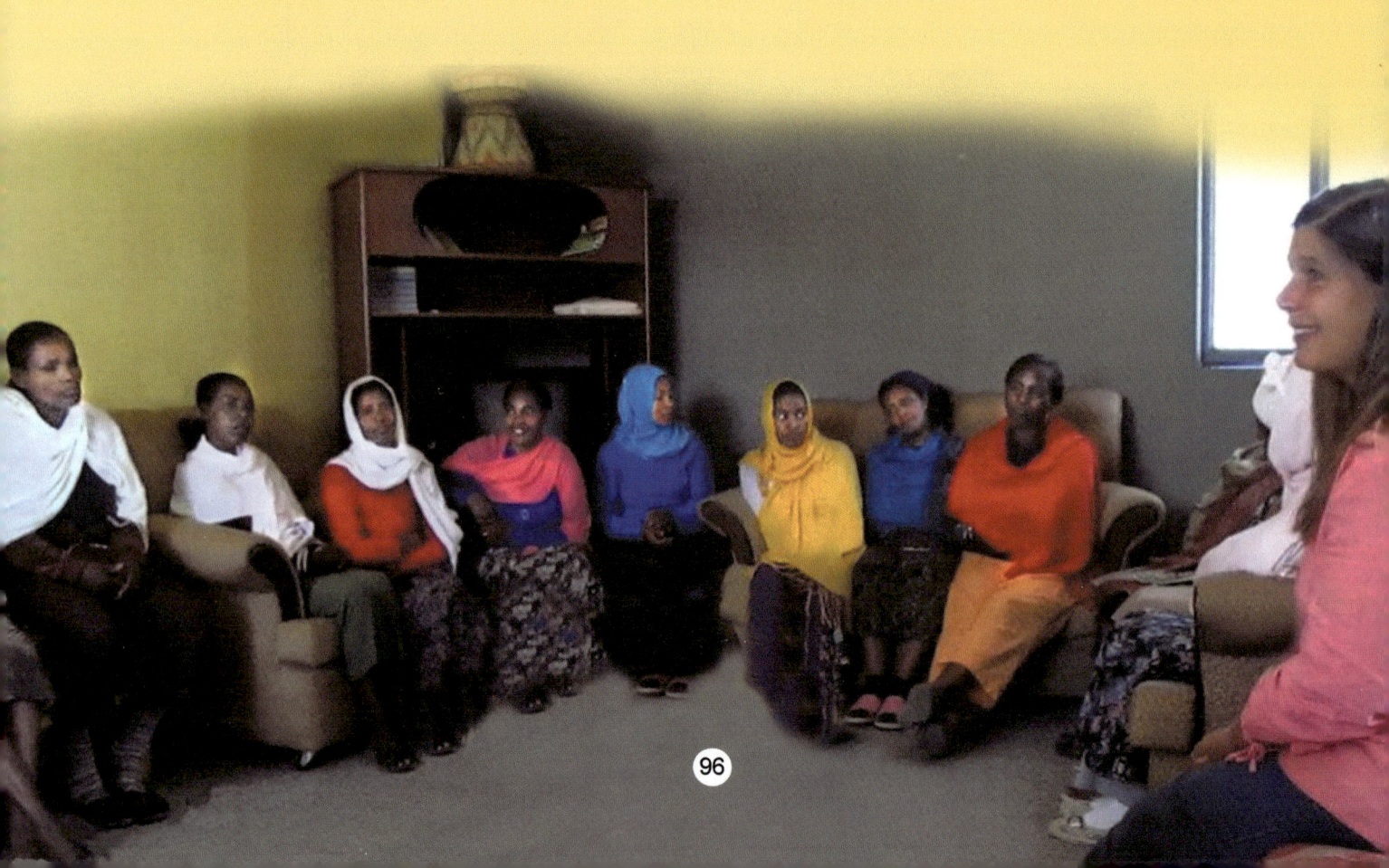